Professionalism, Work, and Clinical Responsibility in Pharmacy

David J. Tipton, PhD

Associate Professor
Mylan School of Pharmacy
Duquesne University
Pittsburgh, Pennsylvania

D1532598

JONES & BARTLETT
LEARNING

World Headquarters
Jones & Bartlett Learning
5 Wall Street
Burlington, MA 01803
978-443-5000
info@jblearning.com
www.jblearning.com

Jones & Bartlett Learning books and products are available through most bookstores and online booksellers. To contact Jones & Bartlett Learning directly, call 800-832-0034, fax 978-443-8000, or visit our website, www.jblearning.com.

Professionalism, Work, and Clinical Responsibility in Pharmacy is an independent publication and has not been authorized, sponsored, or otherwise approved by the owners of the trademarks or service marks referenced in this product.

Some images in this book feature models. These models do not necessarily endorse, represent, or participate in the activities represented in the images.

This publication is designed to provide accurate and authoritative information in regard to the Subject Matter covered. It is sold with the understanding that the publisher is not engaged in rendering legal, accounting, or other professional service. If legal advice or other expert assistance is required, the service of a competent professional person should be sought.

Production Credits

Publisher: William Brottmiller
Senior Acquisitions Editor: Katey Birtcher
Associate Editor: Teresa Reilly
Production Manager: Julie Champagne Bolduc
Production Assistant: Stephanie Rineman
Marketing Manager: Grace Richards
VP, Manufacturing and Inventory Control:
   Therese Connell
Composition: Lapiz, Inc.
Cover Design: Karen LeDuc and Kristin E. Parker
Cover and Title Page Image: © Andrija Markovic/
   ShutterStock, Inc.
Printing and Binding: Edwards Brothers Malloy
Cover Printing: Edwards Brothers Malloy

To order this product, use ISBN: 978-1-284-02206-3

Library of Congress Cataloging-in-Publication Data

Tipton, David J., 1948-
    Professionalism, work, and clinical responsibility in pharmacy / by David J. Tipton.
       p. ; cm.
    Includes bibliographical references and index.
    ISBN 978-1-4496-5743-7 -- ISBN 1-4496-5743-5
    I. Title.
    [DNLM: 1. Pharmacy. 2. Professional Competence. QV 21]
    615.1--dc23
                                                                    2012046661

6048

Printed in the United States of America
17 16 15 14 13   10 9 8 7 6 5 4 3 2 1

Contents

CHAPTER 4 | 43
Self-Awareness

CHAPTER 5 | 61
Self-Management

CHAPTER 6 | 73
Social Awareness

Introduction

THIS IS A BOOK IN layers. The first layer focuses on emotional intelligence. Emotional intelligence is your ability to understand your emotions and the emotions of another person, and then craft a behavior based on these emotions that is appropriate to the context. Emotional intelligence is not about suppressing or indulging emotions; it is about using emotions to accomplish personal and organizational goals—in this case, acting professionally in both your work role and your clinical role. There are four aspects of emotional intelligence: self-awareness, self-management, social awareness, and relationship management.

The second layer focuses on professionalism. The American Board of Internal Medicine model of professionalism is used. The model consists of six attributes: altruism, accountability, duty, excellence, honor and integrity, and respect for others.

The third layer relates the concept of emotional intelligence to professionalism. The connection is made by asking you to consider the following questions:

Self-awareness: What are my values, attitudes, beliefs, feelings, and behaviors in regard to altruism, accountability, duty, excellence, honor, integrity, and respect for others?

Self-management: How do I manage myself regarding the professional obligations of altruism, accountability, duty, excellence, honor, integrity, and respect for others?

Social awareness: How do I use social awareness to facilitate altruism, accountability, duty, excellence, honor, integrity, and respect for others?

Relationship management: How do I manage my relationships to reflect altruism, accountability, duty, excellence, honor, integrity, and respect for others?

Having merged the ideas of emotional intelligence and professionalism, both frameworks are applied to clinical responsibility. The topics discussed are expertise and thinking; emotional labor, compassion fatigue, stress, and burnout; establishing credibility; worry, fear, and errors; and interprofessional relationships.

The frameworks of emotional intelligence and professionalism are applied to work-related issues in the fourth layer of the book. This section considers bosses; careers; difficult conversations; new supervisors; politics; romantic relationships at work; and, trust, delegation, empowerment. This section concludes with practical advice on these issues.

The book is organized into parts based on these four layers: Part I focuses on emotional intelligence; Part II is devoted to professionalism; Part III looks at clinical responsibility; and Part IV deals with work-related issues.

Most chapters are short. Topics are presented primarily in a question and answer format with minimal footnoting. Each chapter contains exercises and discussion points, and is written with the understanding that pharmacy students are busy.

Each chapter attempts to convey the best that the literature has to offer on the topic being discussed. By design this is not a complete review of the often extensive writing and thinking on these points. Pharmacy students simply do not have the time for such detail.

The core learning strategy utilized is self-directed learning operationalized as a personal learning program. What does this mean? It doesn't make sense to say to a student, "Here is a white coat, be a professional." More appropriately, a formal, self-directed, personalized, targeted, incremental, "small wins" approach to professional enhancement, clinical responsibility, and work is used. For a topic such as altruism, students will determine what aspect of this element of professionalism is most important to them and then develop their own unique approach to its enhancement. Several years ago it became acceptable to sing the national anthem in various styles. The words and sentiments were always the same, but the rhythm and delivery varied by artist. The methodology used to enhance professionalism will be the same for each student, but the specific issue and program will vary by student.

As a new graduate, you will arrive for your first day of work. Your employer will have expectations of you including, among other things, that you are clinically adept, organizationally effective, financially aware, customer oriented, managerially skilled, and inter- and intrapersonally competent. In addition, they will expect you to conduct yourself as a professional.

This book is designed to help you use emotional intelligence to meet your clinical responsibilities and become an ethical, responsible professional who contributes to the overall success of your workplace.

Finally, in choosing a career and a college experience, students are confronted with two choices. One is to choose a career with tangible economic prospects at the end of college. Pharmacy surely meets this test. Unfortunately, in making the choice to become a pharmacist, students are denied some of the freedom to pursue courses of study that offer significant opportunities for personal growth. It is an unfortunate by-product of the rigor demanded in becoming a pharmacist. As a result, some pharmacy students may feel deficient in some of the skills, attitudes, and behaviors that make for a successful life. This book is a small attempt to address this gap.

Acknowledgments

IMPOSSIBLE AS IT SEEMS TO me, I graduated from pharmacy school more than 40 years ago. For some reason, I was not apprehensive about what, at the time, passed for clinical activities. I knew I didn't have to know the answer to every question. I knew I would be able to find the answer and formulate a response. I knew I could process the orders and was comfortable in dealing with the patients. What did frighten me, in an inarticulate, but nevertheless sensed way, was that I didn't know how things worked, how things got done. I knew I would now be competing—not with 23-year-old classmates, but with practitioners with 30, 40, or 50 years of experience.

Hopefully, the reader senses that this is a book not only about professionalism, clinical responsibility, and work, but also about how things work, how things get done. While the topics might not be express instructions on accomplishing things, they touch on the personal, intangible aspects of self and others that facilitate accomplishment and productivity.

Many thanks to my collaborators, Dr. Thomas Mattei, Dr. Vincent Giannetti, and Dr. Michael Shaner—colleagues, mentors, and friends all. Also, thanks to Drs. Kurt Wolfgang and Randy Tomko for taking time to share their perspectives on these topics.

Finally, to my wife, Michele, for tolerating my distracted presence, and to my sons, Matt, Scott, and Joe. This book is for all of you in more ways than you can imagine.

Contributor

Vincent Giannetti, PhD
Professor of Pharmaceutical Administration
Mylan School of Pharmacy
Division of Clinical, Social, and Administrative Sciences
Duquesne University
Pittsburgh, Pennsylvania

Reviewers

Michael C. Berger, PharmD, BCPS
Clinical Assistant Professor
University of Kentucky College of Pharmacy
Lexington, Kentucky

Anthony Corigliano, RPh
Assistant Professor of Pharmacy Practice/Laboratory Coordinator
Wegmans School of Pharmacy
St. John Fisher College
Rochester, New York

Steven J. Crosby, BSP, RPh, MA, FASCP
Assistant Professor of Pharmacy Practice
Department of Pharmacy Practice
Massachusetts College of Pharmacy and Health Sciences
Boston, Massachusetts

Natalie A. DiPietro, PharmD, MPH
Assistant Professor of Pharmacy Practice
Raabe College of Pharmacy
Ohio Northern University
Ada, Ohio

Jason Glowczewski, PharmD, MBA
Manager, Pharmacy and Oncology
University Hospitals Geauga Medical Center
Affiliate Assistant Professor of Pharmacy Practice
University of Findlay
Lyndhurst, Ohio

Paul J. Oesterman, PharmD
Associate Professor of Pharmacy Practice
Roseman University of Health Sciences
Adjunct Faculty
College of Osteopathic Medicine
Touro University Nevada
Henderson, Nevada

Jason Perepelkin, BA, BComm, MSc, PhD
Assistant Professor of Social and Administrative Pharmacy
University of Saskatchewan
Saskatoon, Saskatchewan, Canada

Melissa Ruminski, PharmD
University Hospitals Geauga Medical Center
Chardon, Ohio

PART I

Emotional Intelligence

Ask yourself:

> If I were more self-aware would I be a better practitioner, more clinically adept, a more productive professional?

> If I could manage myself better would I be a better practitioner, more clinically adept, a more productive professional?

> If I were more socially aware would I be a better practitioner, more clinically adept, a more productive professional?

> If I managed my relationships better would I be a better practitioner, more clinically adept, a more productive professional?

The answer to each of these questions must be an unequivocal yes. Taken together, each of these personal aspects—self-awareness, self-management, social awareness, and relationship management—constitutes emotional intelligence. This section focuses on increasing your level of emotional intelligence for the express purpose of increasing your professionalism, elevating your understanding of your clinical responsibilities, and making you a more productive and effective practitioner at work.

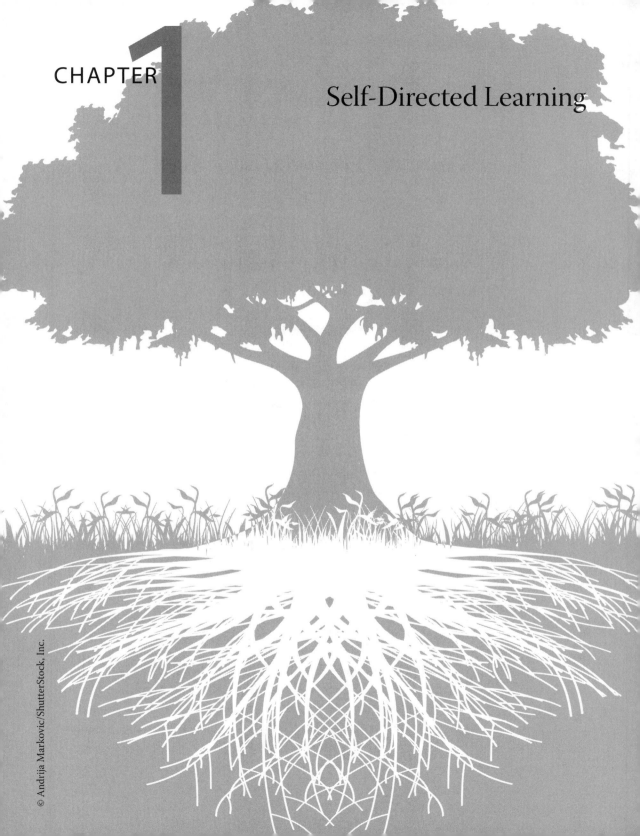

CHAPTER

1

Self-Directed Learning

© Andrija Markovic/ShutterStock, Inc.

✦ DESIRED EDUCATIONAL OUTCOME

- List the concepts related to self-directed learning.

✦ DESIRED PERSONAL OUTCOME

- Become adept at self-directed learning and developing personal learning plans.

What's the Typical Approach to Pharmacy Education?

IN THE FAMILIAR WAYS, SCHOOLS of pharmacy train students to assimilate and recall specific facts, calculate correct answers, and demonstrate mastery of specific skills and techniques. Schools of pharmacy can also train students to demonstrate clinical judgment and problem solving. The approach used to do this, at most schools, is termed *pedagogy*. Pedagogy is the art and science of teaching children. (This is not to demean students; it simply reflects the definition and what actually goes on.) This approach assumes that students have dependent personalities, learning is subject motivated, motivation is extrinsic, and prior experience is not relevant. The extrinsic motivation for this process is the carrot of a degree and licensure. Obtaining licensure is no small thing. For the acquisition of the technical and procedural aspects of pharmacy this approach is time honored and reasonably effective, especially if licensure is the primary objective. However, as a practical matter, relatively little of this information is retained for significant amounts of time.

What Happens as Students Age?

AT 23–25 YEARS OF AGE, most pharmacy students are taking on the characteristics of adult learners. Educating adult learners requires different assumptions and a different approach to instruction. That approach is termed *andragogy*—the art and science of helping adults learn. The assumptions for adult learners are (adapted from Taylor & Kroth, 2009):

- *Self-concept:* As a person matures they move from being a dependent personality to being self-directed. As such, anything that is viewed as being forced on them will be resisted.

- *Experience:* As a person matures they have a backlog of experiences. These experiences are a resource for learning.

- *Readiness to learn:* As a person matures, readiness to learn is a function of the perceived relevance of the topic.

- *Orientation to learn:* Adults learn those things that will help them solve a problem in real life.

- *Motivation to learn:* With maturity, internal motivation is the key to learning.

- *The need to know:* With maturity, people need to know why they need to know something.

Accepting that these assumptions apply to pharmacy students, the approach to their education should reflect these assumptions.

What's the Best Way to Enhance Professionalism?

NOTE THAT IN THIS SECTION we use the term *professionalism* as an umbrella term for emotional intelligence, professionalism, clinical responsibility, and work. The same technique of self-directed learning will be applied to each of these areas.

If the educational approaches that worked earlier in their careers will not work, and recognizing that educating for professionalism differs from the typical pharmacy topics, then what is the best approach? The following are critical steps in professional education:

- To borrow from the book *The Lessons of Experience* on the development of managers, "The primary responsibility for effective management development resides in the managers themselves" (McCall,

1988, p. x). The author terms this fact the "gut truth." It is possible for a pharmacy student to have the academic prowess to master the curriculum, complete clinical rotations, and pass the boards without ever addressing any deficiencies in professionalism, as long as they meet some minimal standard. The "gut truth" is that legitimate professional growth will be up to the student.

- Next is a change in mindset. If you don't think professionalism can be increased then you see it as a fixed aspect of yourself, like your height. If you think professionalism can be increased then you see it as akin to increasing the size of a muscle—all you need to do is exercise.

- Goals come in two varieties. One goal is a performance goal, that is, to get the required grade to pass any formal course. A second and more powerful goal is a learning goal, to actually learn the material and become a professional.

- No two students will need to improve their professional development in exactly the same way. Students will be deficient in both kind and degree of professional behavior. Thus, a one-size-fits-all approach to professional development won't work. As young adults, students will learn only what they want to learn. Under coercion, any behavioral changes shown will quickly be extinguished. Sustainable personal change endures only if the individual wants it to. Self-directed change is intentional and conscious, a progression from who you are to who you want to be (Boyatzis, 2002). Self-directed learners are characterized as curious, motivated, disciplined, methodical, reflective, self-aware, persistent, responsible, and self-sufficient with highly developed information-seeking skills and critical thinking abilities (Litzinger, Wise, & Lee, 2005).

- Not all students learn in the same manner. Some students' professional behavior may be altered by association with a colleague, others will need to read something, and others may need to talk to someone. How something is learned doesn't matter. What needs to be understood is that each student will vary in how they do it. Further, some students may get the "picture" almost overnight, whereas some may take years. The point is that all students are different, and their learning styles and capacities vary.

(•) Mastering professionalism is painful. Nothing worthwhile is ever acquired without effort. Effort gives meaning to our lives. This task is just like acquiring clinical expertise—if it were easy everybody and anybody would do it. Think of any skill you have acquired in your life: a sweet golf swing, learning to play an instrument, riding a bike, organic chemistry. When asked the best way to get to Carnegie Hall, the musician replied, "Practice." Being a professional requires practice. You have to be willing to lean into the discomfort. "Learning to become an effective self-directed learner is probably the greatest intellectual and psychological challenge that an individual can face in a lifetime" (Dealtry, 2004, p. 108).

• There is no express elevator to the pinnacle of professionalism. It requires commitment to a process of gradual improvement. Think of how a foreign language is mastered. Day after day, vocabulary, idioms, grammar, and the rules of syntax are acquired. Professionalism is similar. Gradually, the attitudes, values, and behaviors that constitute professionalism are recognized, understood, assimilated, and then woven into the pattern of our practice. No one loses 100 pounds in a day; people lose 1 pound 100 times over an extended period. Small wins in the pursuit of professionalism are the order of the day.

• No one is ever completely and consistently or perfectly professional. There is always something more to be learned. The pursuit of professionalism is like an asymptote in algebra. An asymptote is a curve that approaches, but never touches, a straight line. On your last day of work, 40–50 years in the future, there will be some aspect of your professionalism that can be improved. Professionalism is not a dichotomous variable (either/or) but a continuous variable (more/less).

In summary:

• Legitimate professional growth is up to the student.
• Alter your mindset to recognize that professionalism can change.
• Establish mastery as a goal.
• Recognize you will direct your own program of professional growth.
• Determine the best way for you to learn.

- Lean into the discomfort.
- Small wins are the order of the day.
- Understand that you will never be perfect at this.

Personal change is hard. Think of the times in your life you vowed to improve some aspect of your behavior—study more, eat better, exercise more. Consider the outcomes. To be more emotionally intelligent and more professional is to engage in personal change. Telling a student to be more professional, be more self-aware, read this code of conduct, or attend this seminar doesn't work. Hard as they might be, mastering the typical pharmacy school theories, concepts, and techniques are nothing compared to the task of mastering yourself and creating your professional identity.

What Are the Mechanics of Enhancing Professionalism?

ENHANCING PROFESSIONALISM IS AN EXERCISE in self-science and can be thought of as a self-oriented and self-directed experiment. As such, it helps students to think of themselves as laboratory rats. Imagine looking down on yourself, as if you are in a maze. What are my tendencies and patterns, when do they emerge, what are the circumstances, with whom do they emerge, what am I feeling, what am I thinking, what is happening with my body, and so on? Essentially, you are trying to develop an objective database that captures your modus operandi for navigating the world around you. It is from this self database that a personal professionalism project emerges. Feedback of any type is a rich source of information in developing this personal database.

From this personal database, one can begin to formulate an area of professionalism for enhancement. A key consideration in developing these plans is that the aspect for professional enhancement be as targeted as possible. Time and care must be spent in sharpening the focus. For a particular student, the general area may be linked to relationships with others. To make it more specific, the student focuses on a tendency to anger when under stress and the potential harm to relationships. More specifically, she could focus on the anger associated with long lines at the drive-up window, or even more focused, the anger at the long lines on a night before an exam and the way this anger clouds her relationship with an older, female, high school–educated technician. Think of this process as an inverted funnel moving from the general to the specific. This approach is analogous to developing any good scientific experiment in that developing a focused, testable hypothesis is key. Thus, a student may undertake to understand what causes technicians in the circumstances just described to lose their composure. This is a long way from saying "be more professional."

The mechanics of enhancing professionalism center on developing a personal learning plan. The essence of a personal learning plan is that the student self-identifies that aspect of professionalism they want to address. The student then identifies and implements unique activities and develops or acquires products and resources to address their particular issue. Next, the type of evidence that will be used to determine whether goals have been met are declared. Finally, a timeline for completion is determined. Once the process has been completed, the student should reflect on the process and the outcome. A personal learning plan format is presented here.

Personal Learning Plan: Professionalism

THESE STEPS CAN BE COMPILED on a single page containing the following:

What prompted me to develop this plan?

What is the general area for improvement?

What is the specific issue for improvement?

Why is this important to me?

How do I generally act in these areas?

What are my goals?

What prompted this effort?

What strategies are required?

Who/what is necessary to meet my goals with this strategy?

How will I measure the success/failure of this effort?

How long will I focus on this effort?

How will I reflect and capture a lesson from this effort that can be generalized to other circumstances?

EXERCISES

⫸ Self-Directed Learning Readiness Scale

Please record your response for each question using the following scale:
1 = strongly disagree; 2 = disagree; 3 = neither agree nor disagree; 4 = agree;
5 = strongly agree

1. I solve problems using a plan. _____

2. I prioritize my work. _____

3. I like to solve (answer) puzzles/questions. _____

4. I manage my time well. _____

5. I have good management skills. _____

6. I set strict time frames. _____

7. I prefer to plan my own learning. _____

8. I prefer to direct my own learning. _____

9. I believe the role of the teacher is to act as a resource person. _____

10. I am systematic in my learning. _____

11. I am able to focus on a problem. _____

12. I often review the way pharmacy practices are conducted. _____

13. I need to know why. _____

14. I critically evaluate new ideas. _____

15. I prefer to set my own learning goals. _____

Higher scores indicate a higher level of readiness for self-directed learning.

Source: Fisher, M., King, J., & Tague, G. (2001). Development of a self-directed learning readiness scale for nursing education. *Nurse Education Today, 21,* 516–525.

⫸ Identifying Areas for Enhancing Professionalism

For some students, determining an area for professional growth and developing the process may be difficult. Several methods for making this determination are presented here.

Boyatzis' Theory of Self-Directed Learning

Discovery No. 1: My Ideal Self: Who do I want to be?

Discovery No. 2: My Real Self: Who am I?

Strengths: Where are my ideal and real selfs similar?

Gaps: Where are my ideal and real selfs different?

Discovery No. 3: My learning agenda—building on my strengths while reducing gaps.

Discovery No. 4: New behavior, thoughts, and feelings through experimentation. Creating and building new neural pathways through practicing to mastery.

The key aspect of this model is to recognize the gaps, or deficiencies, in where you are and where you want to be.

Source: Adapted from Boyatzis, R. E. (2002). Unleashing the power of self-directed learning. In Ronald R. Sims (Ed.), *Changing the way we manage change: The consultants speak* (pp. 13–32). Westport, CT: Quorum.

⫸ Emotional Intelligence Framework

Emotions convey information about ourselves and the world. Emotional intelligence is the ability to understand our emotions and those of another person, and then craft an effective behavior appropriate to the task. Tuning in to our emotional world and the emotional world of others spotlights areas for professional growth. Methods for highlighting areas for professional growth using emotional intelligence are suggested here.

Strongest emotional reaction: Identify the strongest emotional reaction you have experienced during school, on rotations, or at work. Describe the context, the circumstances, the people involved, what you were feeling, how you behaved, and the outcome.

Hot buttons: What circumstances, activities, and people cause you to lose your composure? The times that you "lost it" are areas for professional growth.

Fears: Think of the aspects of practice that frighten you.

The key assumption with this approach is that any area that elicits a strong emotional reaction or frightens you is a fertile area for exploration and improvement.

⚬ Appreciative Inquiry

Appreciative inquiry is based on the recognition that all of us are particularly good at something, and what we focus on becomes our reality. Focusing on our deficiencies becomes our reality. In contrast, asking questions of ourselves highlights what we are good at. We then spend more of our effort in doing this, rather than attempting to correct deficiencies. So, how do you get better if you only focus on what you are good at? Recognizing you are good at certain things helps you develop the confidence and comfort to move to areas for improvement. Anchored in the knowledge that you are good at something, you can bring more of the same to areas you want to strengthen.

Appreciative inquiry questions:

1. Think of an aspect of professionalism that is a strength, something you are good at and noted for by others.

2. Think of a current situation involving your professional behavior, and consider a new way of perceiving it.
   a. What is good about this situation, what can I appreciate?
   b. What do I really want?
   c. What am I focusing on? Can I shift my focus?
   d. What learning is available to me, and how can I open up to it?

This approach asks you to consider things you are good at and then extend and leverage those strengths to other areas.

Source: Adapted from Kelm, J. B. (2005). *Appreciative living.* Wake Forest, NC: Venet.

ᐧᕽᐧᕽᐧᕽ Learning History

Adult education assumes that as a person matures they have a backlog of experiences. These experiences are a resource for learning. The question is how to record these experiences and then access the relevant lessons. A personal learning history accomplishes this task. The process of writing a personal learning history is simple. First, on a piece of paper create a two-column table. In the left column record a narrative, the story of what happened; for example, the story of your first clinical rotation. Write the story from your perspective; however, if you are aware of other people's points of view, incorporate these also. In the right column analyze what happened, looking for patterns and areas for improvement. The material in the right column becomes the focus of your personal learning plan. Having someone else read your learning history will confirm the validity of your interpretation of events.

ᐧᕽᐧᕽᐧᕽ Critical Incident Reports

A refinement of the learning history is the development of a critical incident report and reflection on its meaning. A critical incident report is a short, narrative story of a specific event you judge to have significant importance in your professional development. A critical incident can be a learning experience, a challenging occurrence, a personally influential event, or something you witnessed. In developing these reports, think of yourself as a Monday morning quarterback critiquing your performance for the past week. Capturing the incident is the first part of the process; reflection on the meaning of these incidents is also required.

Describe an incident that was particularly meaningful to you.

Describe a professional relationship that was particularly meaningful to you.

Describe a patient relationship that was particularly meaningful to you.

Based on your responses to the exercises, write a one-paragraph description of yourself as it relates to self-directed learning.

◈ WHAT'S IMPORTANT TO YOU IN THIS CHAPTER?

With several of your classmates, discuss the idea or ideas that are most likely to be helpful to you in developing a self-directed learning program for yourself.

◈ REFERENCES

Boyatzis, R. E. (2002). Unleashing the power of self-directed learning. In Ronald R. Sims (Ed.), *Changing the way we manage change: The consultants speak* (pp. 13–32). Westport, CT: Quorum.

Dealtry, R. (2004). Professional practice: The savvy learner. *Journal of Workplace Learning, 16*, 101–109.

Fisher, M., King, J., & Tague, G. (2001). Development of a self-directed learning readiness scale for nursing education. *Nurse Education Today, 21*, 516–525.

Litzinger, T. A., Wise, J. C., & Lee, S. H. (2005). Self-directed learning readiness among engineering undergraduate students. *Journal of Engineering Education, 94*(2), 215–221.

McCall, Jr., M. W., Lombardo, M. M., & Morrison, A. M. (1988). *The lessons of experience.* Lexington, MA: Lexington.

Taylor, B., & Kroth, M. (2009). Andragogy's transition into the future: Meta-analysis of andragogy and its search for a measureable instrument. *Journal of Adult Education, 38*(1), 11.

◈ SUGGESTED READINGS

Amabile, T. M., & Kramer, S. J. (2011, May). The power of small wins. *Harvard Business Review*, 71–80.

Branch, W. T. (2005). Use of critical incident reports in medical education. *Journal of General Internal Medicine, 20*, 1063–1067.

Challis, M. (2000). AMEE medical education guide no. 19: Personal learning plans. *Medical Teacher, 22*(3), 225–236.

Chan, S. (2010). Applications of andragogy in multi-disciplined teaching and learning. *Journal of Adult Education, 39*(2), 25–35.

Dweck, C. S. (2000). *Self-theories.* New York, NY: Taylor and Francis.

Dweck, C. S. (2006). *Mindset.* New York, NY: Ballantine.

Gardner, H. (2006). *Changing minds.* Boston, MA: Harvard Business School Press.

Glasser, W. (1976). *Positive addiction.* New York, NY: Harper and Row.

Hammond, S. A. (1998). *Appreciative inquiry.* Bend, OR: Thin.

Hilliard, C. (2006). Using structured reflection on a critical incident to develop a professional portfolio. *Nursing Standard, 21*(2), 35–40.

Kelm, J. B. (2005). *Appreciative living.* Wake Forest, NC: Venet.

Kleiner, A., & Roth, G. (1997, September–October). How to make experience your company's best teacher. *Harvard Business Review,* 172–177.

May, N., Becker, D., Frankel, R., Hazlip, J., Harmon, R., Plews-Ogan, M., Schorling, J., Williams, A., & Whitney, D. (2011). *Appreciative inquiry in healthcare.* Brunswick, OH: Crown Custom.

Seligman, M. E. P. (2007). *What you can change . . . and what you can't.* New York, NY: Vintage.

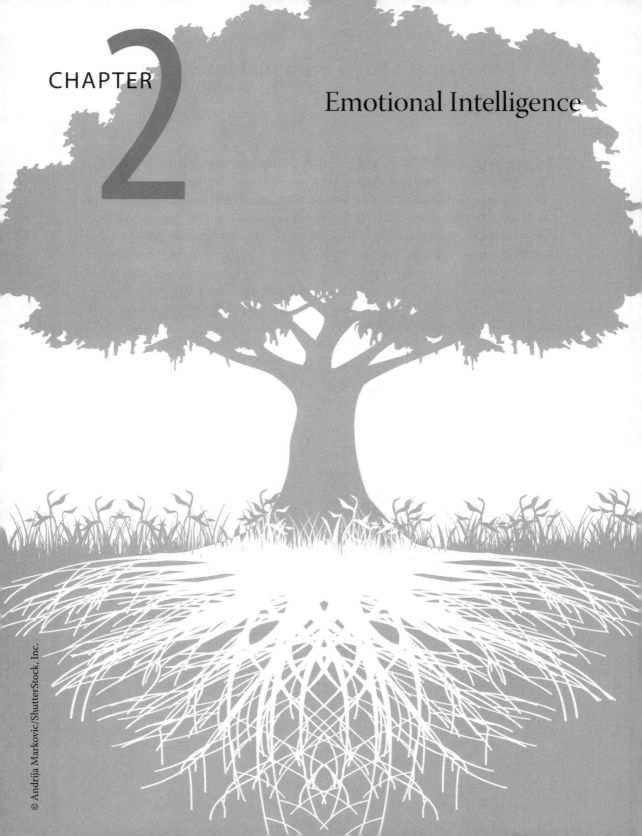

CHAPTER

2

Emotional Intelligence

Pre-Assessment: Emotional Intelligence

Mind Mapping

Consider the term below. Without thinking or editing, write down the ideas, concepts, examples, contradictions, and theories that come to mind. Do not array them in any systematic or orderly manner. Scatter them about the page. Now, draw lines between your additions, indicating that there is a relationship between the terms. If something causes something else, indicate this with an arrow. Relationships may be reciprocal—both cause each other—requiring arrows at both ends. Indicate the strength of the relationship by darkening and thickening the lines; stronger relationships have darker and thicker lines. Most important: There is no right answer. Do not compare with your classmates. What you have is a mind map, your mental representation of the topic. Review to determine if anything has changed following this chapter.

Emotional intelligence

⟨⟩ DESIRED EDUCATIONAL OUTCOMES

- Describe emotional intelligence.
- Describe the four domains of emotional intelligence.
- Discuss emotional hijackings.
- Discuss why emotional intelligence is important.

⟨⟩ DESIRED PERSONAL OUTCOME

- Acquire an enhanced personal level of emotional intelligence.

What Is Emotional Intelligence?

EMOTIONAL INTELLIGENCE IS THE ABILITY to understand your own and other people's emotions, and craft a functional behavior that is suitable to the context. Emotional intelligence does not require that emotions be suppressed or denied; rather, emotions are used to achieve objectives. Some people are better at understanding themselves and the needs of others, and building successful and productive relationships. These people are emotionally intelligent. Emotional intelligence is the social lubrication that facilitates relationships between people.

The idea of emotional intelligence emerged from research on multiple intelligences suggesting that people vary not just in their cognitive abilities, the traditional idea of intelligence, but also on other dimensions, such as musical, spatial, kinesthetic, and intra- and interpersonal understanding.

Whether it is really intelligence or actually a skill that can be learned is debatable. For our purposes, emotional intelligence is viewed as a skill. From this perspective, levels of emotional intelligence are not fixed, but can be improved on.

What Are the Domains of Emotional Intelligence?

EMOTIONAL INTELLIGENCE HAS FOUR DOMAINS or core skills: self-awareness, self-management, social awareness, and relationship management. The first two skills, self-awareness and self-management, are primarily about the individual; they are internal. The second two skills, social awareness and relationship management, are about the individual's relationship to the world; they are external.

What Is Self-Awareness?

Self-awareness is the ability to understand who you are. What are your tendencies; what are your emotional reactions to certain circumstances? What type of people upset you? Which challenges energize you, and which intimidate you? What are you afraid of? The potential number of things you can learn about yourself is unlimited, as experience reveals unfathomed aspects of yourself. The level of self-awareness that is appropriate does not require plumbing the inner depths of your soul and subconscious. Instead, ask yourself in an objective way: Do you understand how you operate in the world? Self-awareness is the foundation on which other aspects of emotional intelligence are built.

What Is Self-Management?

Self-management is what you do, or do not do, that is appropriate to the context. Context is key. Behaviors appropriate to a student graduation party are ill-advised at a company Christmas party. Self-management requires monitoring your behaviors in specific, discrete circumstances as well as your entrenched tendencies. Self-management requires sublimating your immediate emotional needs for your longer term success. It is difficult to react appropriately in all circumstances; often you will get it wrong. Effective self-management requires self-correction, the quicker the better. A self-managed person is the CEO of the self.

What Is Social Awareness?

Social awareness requires paying attention to the people and the world around you. You have to look and listen—effectively. This requires that you stop talking and stop listening to the internal dialogue in your head. Social intelligence requires seeing people as they are, not as you would like them to be. There is a tendency for all of us to seek confirmation of our own internal beliefs. We do this by focusing on the things that confirm our beliefs and ignoring disconfirming information. Socially aware people understand this bias and understand "it is what it is."

What Is Relationship Management?

We all live in the shadow of one another. Relationships are the key to everything. Relationship management builds on the three other emotional intelligence domains. Relationships build over time and take work. They require give and take. Relationship management is a delicate balance between doing things to preserve the relationship and doing things to preserve personal integrity.

What Are Emotional Hijackings?

EMOTIONAL HIJACKINGS, OR FLASHPOINTS, ARE circumstances, people, or objects that provoke uncontrolled emotional reactions. Road rage following being cut off in traffic exemplifies an emotional hijacking. Lashing out at someone if you feel belittled is another example. For some, a spider on the wall elicits panic and fear out of proportion to the threat. Emotional hijackings, or reacting without thinking, can be considered a form of emotional *unintelligence.* A significant aspect of emotional intelligence is understanding and managing emotional hijackings.

Why Is Emotional Intelligence Important?

IN THEIR BOOK *EMOTIONAL INTELLIGENCE 2.0*, Bradberry and Greaves (2009) report the following findings:

- Ninety percent of high performers in their jobs are also high in emotional intelligence.
- Just 20 percent of low performers at work are high in emotional intelligence.
- Emotional intelligence is the single largest predictor of success at work.
- Those high in emotional intelligence, on average, earn $29,000 more than those low in emotional intelligence.

These findings hold true across all industries, at all levels, and in all countries of the world. These results are based on a sample of more than 500,000 individuals. The results speak for themselves regarding the impact of emotional intelligence on career trajectory.

If these results are not sufficient to impress upon you the impact of emotional intelligence, consider the following. As a pharmacy student, you have self-selected and been selected into a group of individuals who on average have an IQ in the neighborhood of 120. In other words, everyone in pharmacy school is smart. Essentially, there is no significant variance in the intelligence level of pharmacy students. What's left to predict career success: emotional intelligence. Thirty years from now those students highest in emotional intelligence will sit at the top of the career ladder, whereas those less self-aware, unable to manage their emotions, who have difficulty reading social situations, and are ill adept at relationships will be working for their classmates. We acknowledge there is individual variation in this prediction, but on average it will hold true.

What Are Some Examples of Emotional Intelligence?

THE FOLLOWING SITUATIONS CAPTURE ASPECTS of emotional intelligence:

- Michael Jordan was cut from his high school basketball team. He used the stigma of this public humiliation to fuel the anger that drove his quest for basketball perfection and success.

- Your 10-year-old son comes home with his first "F" grade on a paper. Rather than lashing out in anger or disappointment, you try to understand his embarrassment and shame. Although not condoning his actions, you discuss the reason for the performance and how to improve while conveying you still love him.

- You witness a large man abusing his 9-year-old daughter in public. You use the anger invoked by this injustice to intervene to protect the child without escalating your response to a personal attack on the abusive father.

Emotional Intelligence at Work

THE FOLLOWING IS A SAMPLE scenario related to emotional intelligence involving RPG (recent pharmacy graduate):

> Having graduated 3 years ago with his Doctor of Pharmacy degree, nothing but good things had happened for RPG. He secured precisely the job he wanted in a major healthcare setting. Each year his responsibilities have increased. His performance has been exemplary on all counts. Coming in to work today, RPG discovered that the technician responsible for mailing IV medications from his department made a mistake in switching mailing labels on two separate orders. Consequently, two patients would receive their medications late. To correct this oversight, both orders had to be reconstituted and delivered overnight at considerable expense. The original orders had to be picked up and destroyed because it was not clear that the required storage conditions had been met. RPG was steaming; he was frightened. His natural inclination was to burst into the department and start yelling, not only at the responsible technician, but at all the staff. In his mind, RPG thought there was no place for subtlety when people's lives were in the balance.

How would you recommend RPG handle the situation?

Assignment: What Do the Practitioners/Others Say?

BE PREPARED TO DISCUSS EMOTIONAL intelligence based on any *one* of the following:

- A discussion with your colleagues, or others, on how they feel and what they know about emotional intelligence
- An article on emotional intelligence, either from the research literature or any other source
- A movie/television program/YouTube video about emotional intelligence
- A book on emotional intelligence (literary, historical, psychological, or any other source)

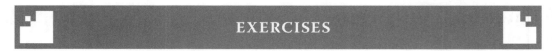

EXERCISES

⫸ How Would You Rate Your Emotional Intelligence?

Ask yourself the following questions, assigning a rating from poor to good. If possible, ask someone else close to you to answer the questions on your behalf. That external perspective will help prevent self-reporting bias. Rate yourself from 1 to 10 on these points, with 1 being poor and 10 being good.

1. How good are you at understanding others from their perspective? _____

2. How sensitive are you about the feelings of others? _____

3. Do you easily make friends? _____

4. Are you willing to express your emotions to others? _____

5. Are you good at solving conflicts? _____

If you (and others) consistently rate you on the high end of the scale, you're lucky: it sounds as if you have a high EQ. If not, you should put some effort into the further development of this crucial part of human functioning.

Source: Kets de Vries, M. (2001). *The leadership mystique.* London: Pearson Education.

⫸ Emotional Type

All of us have a particular style of relating to our emotions and to the world. This is the filter through which we see the world. Understanding our type helps us understand how we behave. Our emotional type is due to inborn temperament and parental influence. No single type is superior to another. Understanding your emotional type is a key element to developing your emotional intelligence. It is a key aspect of self-awareness, but only a beginning. Emotional type can evolve over time. Also, most of us are combinations of several emotional types.

The Intellectual

Intellectuals live in their head. They are cerebral. The world is seen through a rational filter. Intellectuals are at risk of being cut off from their emotions. To determine if you are an intellectual, consider the following:

Do I believe that I can think my way through to any solution?

When presented with a problem, do I immediately start analyzing the pros and cons rather than noticing how I feel?

Am I uncomfortable when people get highly emotional?

Do I tend to get overly serious?

Do I distrust decisions made by the gut?

Do I prefer planning to being spontaneous?

The Empath

Empaths feel everything. They have a finely tuned antenna for emotions. For the empath, intuition is the filter for their world. To determine if you might be an empath, consider the following.

Have I been labeled as too emotional or overly sensitive?

If a friend is distraught, do I feel it too?

Are my feelings easily hurt?

Am I emotionally drained by crowds and require time alone to revive?

Do my nerves get frayed by noise, smells, or excessive talk?

Do I prefer taking my own car places so that I can leave when I please?

Do I overeat to cope with emotional stress?

Am I afraid of becoming engulfed by intimate relationships?

The Rock

Rocks are emotionally strong. They are practical. They are cool. They care about your pain but maintain their boundary. They like life on an even keel but will deal with life's problems. Rocks internalize their emotions. To determine if you are a rock, consider the following:

Is it easier to listen than to share my feelings?

Do I often feel like the most dependable person in the room?

Do people tend to come to me with their troubles?

Am I able to stay calm when others are upset?

Would I rather avoid introspection?

Am I generally satisfied with the status quo in relationships but others are often trying to draw me out emotionally?

The Gusher

Gushers are the opposite of rocks; they are intimately in tune with their emotions and want to share them. They tend to be spontaneous and authentic. Gushers unload stress by verbalizing it. To determine if you are a gusher, consider the following:

> Is it easy for me to express my emotions?
>
> Do I get anxious if I keep my feelings in?
>
> When a problem arises, is my first impulse to pick up the phone?
>
> Do I need to take a poll before finalizing a decision?
>
> Are my friends often telling me, "Too much information"?
>
> Do I have difficulty sensing other people's emotional boundaries?

Source: Adapted from Orloff, J. (2009). *Emotional freedom.* New York, NY: Harmony.

◈ What About the People You Know?

Take a few moments to consider the characteristics of some of the most likeable and not likeable people you have met. Are there patterns in how they conduct themselves? Would you assess one as more emotionally intelligent than the other? How effective are they in their career, their dealings with other people? Note their characteristics in **Table 2.1**.

TABLE 2.1 Characteristics

Likeable Characteristics	Not Likeable Characteristics

◈ What About Famous People?

With several of your classmates, consider people in the news, presidents, celebrities, athletes, and the like. Think of your favorite reality-based program. Which of the people do you consider to be emotionally intelligent?

Based on their public behavior, appearances, and pronouncements, rate their emotional intelligence. Does anyone come to mind that you would rate highly on emotional intelligence? Is there anyone you would rate deficient in emotional intelligence?

_____

_____

_____

⫶ What's the Emotionally Intelligent Thing to Do?

With several of your classmates, discuss the emotionally intelligent response to the following scenarios. Also, consider how not to handle these situations.

The Dinner

You and your fiancée planned a romantic weekend together to celebrate the end of the semester. The only thing left to do before moving and taking the job you want is graduation. The night before leaving you want to go out for dinner. There is considerable disagreement over the restaurant choice. Following a lengthy discussion, you agree to the restaurant your fiancée prefers. Unfortunately, the food, the service, and the ambience are terrible. As you pay the rather expensive bill, you are fuming at the waste of money. What do you advise?

The Grade

You always felt that your preceptor didn't really like you. You are not sure why, but others noticed that the preceptor seemed aloof with you, whereas with other students she was warm and giving. You just received your first evaluation from the preceptor. You were graded as deficient on everything. Even though you had some difficulties, and came to one presentation ill prepared, it was not likely you would be inadequate on all dimensions. You know for a fact that the other clinical staff enjoyed working with you. This evaluation was personally hurtful, the first time something like this has happened to you. It was a stress you did not need. You just found out your mother was going in for tests following a course of treatment for breast cancer. What do you advise?

The Advice

Pharmacy school has been a struggle for you—not because of intellectual deficiencies, but because much of your time was spent on school and national organizations. You served as president of your class, your sorority, and several campus-wide initiatives. You really loved these activities. You took to heart the recommendation that job prospects are enhanced by demonstrating your commitment to the profession and your organizational skills. As a result of these time commitments, you now find yourself in front of the student standing committee petitioning for readmission to the program following your third deficiency. The committee says they will consider reinstatement if you will drop all extracurricular activities and concentrate on academics. You still believe you can do both, it will just take a small adjustment in your time. What do you advise?

Based on your responses to the exercises, write a one-paragraph description of yourself as it relates to emotional intelligence.

✦ WHAT'S IMPORTANT TO YOU IN THE CHAPTER?

With several of your classmates discuss the idea/ideas most likely to effect a change in your values, attitudes, or behaviors. Be succinct—no more than two sentences.

✦ REFERENCES

Bradberry, T., & Greaves, J. (2009). *Emotional intelligence 2.0*. San Diego, CA: Talent Smart.

Kets de Vries, M. (2001). *The leadership mystique*. London: Pearson Education.

Orloff, J. (2009). *Emotional freedom*. New York, NY: Harmony.

⩔ SUGGESTED READINGS

Cherniss, C. (2000, April 15). Emotional intelligence: What it is and why it matters. Presented at the Annual Meeting of the Society for Industrial and Organizational Psychology, New Orleans, LA.

Cote, S., & Miners, C. T. H. (2006). Emotional intelligence, cognitive intelligence, and job performance. *Administrative Science Quarterly*, *51*, 1–28.

Gardner, H. (2004). *Frames of mind: The theory of multiple intelligences.* New York, NY: Basic.

Lynn, A. (2005). *The EQ difference.* New York, NY: Amacom.

Mayer, J. D., Salovey, P., & Caruso, D. R. (2004). A further consideration of the issues of emotional intelligence. *Psychological Inquiry*, *15*(3), 249–255.

Segal, J. (1997). *Raising your emotional intelligence.* New York, NY: Owl.

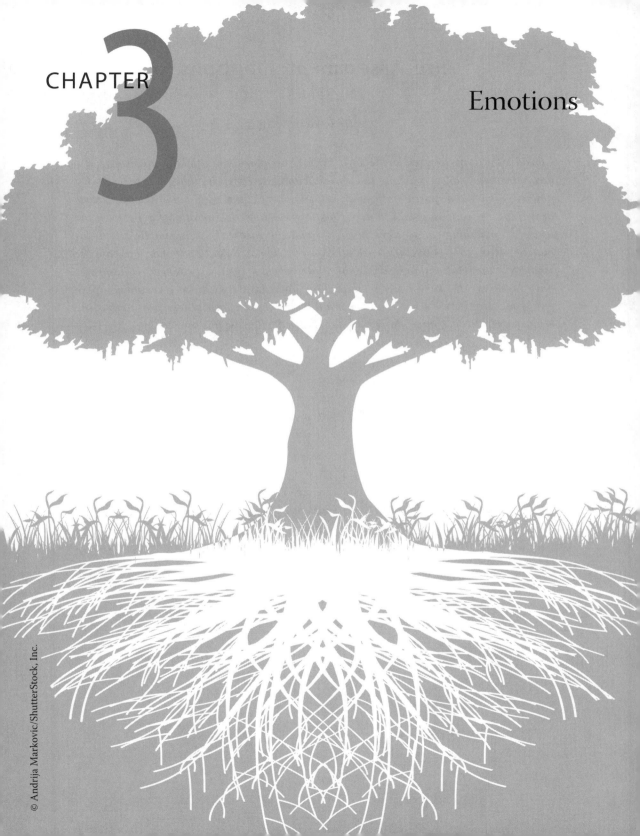

CHAPTER

3

Emotions

Pre-Assessment: Emotions

Mind Mapping

Consider the terms arrayed on the page. For each term, without thinking or editing, write down the ideas, concepts, examples, contradictions, and theories that come to mind. Do not array them in any systematic or orderly manner. Scatter them about the page. Now, draw lines between your additions, indicating that there is a relationship between the terms. If something causes something else, indicate this with an arrow. Relationships may be reciprocal—both cause each other—requiring arrows at both ends. Indicate the strength of the relationship by darkening and thickening the lines; stronger relationships have darker and thicker lines. Most important: There is no right answer. Do not compare with your classmates. *What you have is a mind map, your mental representation of the topic. Review to determine if anything has changed following this chapter.*

Anger
Sadness
Fear
Happiness

⫸ DESIRED EDUCATIONAL OUTCOMES

- Define emotions, mood, and temperament.
- Discuss the myths surrounding emotions.
- Discuss whether you can hide your emotions.

⫸ DESIRED PERSONAL OUTCOME

- Gain an enhanced understanding of your emotional world.

What Are Emotions?

DANIEL GOLEMAN, AUTHOR OF THE book *Emotional Intelligence* (1995), which brought the idea of emotional intelligence to a larger readership, defines an emotion as "... a feeling and its distinctive thoughts, psychological and biological states, and range of propensities to act" (p. 289). Emotions have a cognitive component (thinking), a physiological component (biological), and a behavioral component (acting).

What Are the Primary Emotions?

CERTAIN EMOTIONS (FEAR, ANGER, SADNESS, and enjoyment) are recognized around the world, even by preliterate cultures. The conclusion is that evolution has selected these emotions to be hard-wired into our central nervous system. These four emotions, and their variants, can be blended to create innumerable and subtle emotional shadings. Just as artists see shades and hues of color, emotionally astute individuals can understand and describe the shades and hues of their emotional lives. The following provides an expanded vocabulary of emotions (adapted from Goleman, 1995):

- *Anger:* Fury, outrage, resentment, wrath, exasperation, indignation, vexation, acrimony, animosity, annoyance, irritability, hostility, and at the extreme, pathological hatred and violence
- *Sadness:* Grief, sorrow, cheerlessness, gloom, melancholy, self-pity, loneliness, dejection, despair, and when pathological, severe depression

- *Fear:* Anxiety, apprehension, nervousness, concern, consternation, misgiving, wariness, qualm, edginess, dread, fright, terror, and as a pathology, phobia and panic
- *Enjoyment:* Happiness, joy, relief, contentment, bliss, delight, amusement, pride, sensual pleasure, thrill, rapture, gratification, satisfaction, euphoria, whimsy, ecstasy, and at the extreme, mania

Why Are Some Emotions Hard to Describe?

EMOTIONS CAN BE CLEAN AND simple or multilayered and complex. The anger someone feels in seeing a small child abused is a clean and simple emotion. In contrast, the circumstance of receiving a birthday card from a friend makes you happy, while evoking feelings of guilt because you forgot to send him a card, ultimately giving rise to tinges of anger because he still owes you money. This exemplifies a complex and multilayered emotional response. Another example of a complex emotional reaction is a father looking at his just-born baby; he is ecstatic, but in an instant he becomes alarmed, and then fearful as he realizes there is something wrong with the baby. The circumstance of getting angry because you were angry is another example of a complex and multilayered emotional response. Awareness and learning about emotions require that we develop a nuanced vocabulary of emotions.

Are Emotions Functional?

EACH OF THESE FOUR EMOTIONS has functional and dysfunctional aspects to them. In other words, they can be both beneficial to you and detrimental. For example, anger may motivate you to act, or alienate you from other people; fear will alert you to a threat, or interfere with thinking; sadness may motivate you to reevaluate what you want from life, or inhibit you from taking any action at all; finally, happiness can promote positive relationships, or lead you to unrealistically favorable expectations.

Box 3.1   What Are the Myths Surrounding Emotions?

Certain myths are associated with emotions. On examination, these myths are not supported by logic or neurological studies. The myths include:

- *Emotions are inferior to reason.* Emotions are processed at lower points in the brain; however, emotions are biochemically and structurally intertwined with higher levels of the cortex. Emotions are primitive mechanisms for survival, but also the foundation for creativity, empathy, sociability, and boundless self-knowledge.
- *Emotions are dangerous.* Emotions can be painful, but like physical pain they are signals of deeper pathologies. As warnings, they are indispensible if paid attention to.
- *Self-control is a function of stifling feelings.* Self-control does not come from controlling our feelings, but feeling our feelings.
- *Some emotions are good and others are bad.* Many believe anger is an emotion whose time has passed in our civilized world. But righteous anger associated with injustice is invaluable. All emotions are informative.
- *Emotions cloud your judgment.* It is the mental activity associated with avoiding our emotions that clouds our judgment, not the emotions themselves.

Source: Adapted from Segal, J. (1997). *Raising your emotional intelligence: A practical guide.* New York, NY: Owl.

What Are Moods? What Is Temperament?

EMOTIONS THAT ARE MUTED BUT persist for an extended period (a day or two) are moods; in contrast, the tendency towards a specific mood over a very long time is temperament. For example, I might feel ecstatic for a few moments if someone compliments me, be in a good mood the rest of the day due to the compliment, and stay naturally happy and content for many days at a time because that is my basic disposition or temperament.

What Is the Biology of Emotions?

Poets believe emotions to be intangible. In fact, as neuroscientists know, they are tangible; they are conveyed via biochemical transmitters and recorded in neural pathways. The human brain is an organ whose primary interest is survival. To that end, quick and immediate emotional responses (without thinking) to danger in the environment are useful. Think of the surprise appearance of a snake on a path; the feeling of fear is almost instantaneous. Being quick, these emotional responses are reactionary, often sloppy, and not necessarily completely accurate or appropriate. Emotional responses typically last for only a few seconds before the thinking response kicks in. It is only a small garden snake. No need to panic. The emotional mind reacts to the present as if it were the past. If someone has a bad experience learning to swim she may still have brief moments of fear prior to entering the water, even though she knows how to swim. Or, if a father was loud and abusive to his child, then this child may have brief moments of fear later in life when authority figures arrive.

What is the physiological mechanism for these responses? The senses pick up changes in the environment that are routed initially to the lower brain. At the same time, these sensory changes are routed to the mid-brain, which is the seat of our emotions, via a short and direct pathway, and also to the cerebral cortex, the source of higher order thinking, via a longer pathway. This is why one can have an emotional response without "thinking," such as when someone says, "I was so angry I just lost it." The implication of this is that at least for a brief moment our emotions can be in control causing us to be out of control Our physiology guarantees this. Our physiology also guarantees that by taking a moment or two and allowing the higher elements of our brain to take command we can control our emotions. Emotions operate in the range of our conscious awareness, whereas moods operate at the fringe of our conscious awareness. Finally, some emotional responses are outside the realm of conscious awareness.

What Do I Learn from My Emotions?

Emotions contain data. specifically, emotions contain data about people—you, other people, social situations, and interactions. Emotions provide real-time feedback about what is going on around you.

Can I Ignore My Emotions, or Hide Them?

EMOTIONS AFFECT EVERYTHING YOU DO. You can be mindful of them, you can suppress them, but you can't ignore them. Emotions work in ways not yet completely understood. Even presumably highly rational decision processes are influenced by your emotional state. Positive and negative moods impact how you decide. Many situations demand that you control or suppress your emotions. The simple fact is that although you can sometimes camouflage your emotions, with more regularity than you suppose, some people read your emotions regularly and all people read your emotions occasionally.

Why Do I Always React the Same Way?

IF ADDICTION IS DEFINED AS something you can't stop, then each of us is addicted to our emotions. Every morning, we all get up and put on our own familiar and comfortable emotional coat. Even though the emotion may be negative and not self-serving, it is the one we choose on a daily basis. This emotional addiction is based on the fact that neurons that fire together create neural networks. These networks reflect the experienced patterns of our emotions, thoughts, and behaviors. This explains why, on a daily basis, you tend to feel like a victim, or slightly sad, or optimistic. This explains why similar situations and people always evoke the same emotional response. There is no rule that says if a driver cuts you off in traffic you must get angry. It is only your neural network responding as it always does to this circumstance. Paradoxically, negative emotions like anger and sadness can be strangely comforting due to their familiarity. Though you might be addicted to specific emotional patterns, you can, with conscious effort, change these patterns.

Emotions at Work

THE FOLLOWING IS A SAMPLE scenario related to emotional intelligence involving RPG (recent pharmacy graduate):

RPG loved the babies. She could hardly wait to get to work each day in the NIC unit. But the work was high stress, demanding all of her clinical faculties. There simply was no room for error when dealing with a human life that came in a 500-gram package. RPG remembered the day the physician turned to her and said, "We have about 20 minutes to dose this baby, or it will die." One of her colleagues recently had miscalculated an insulin dose for a baby by a power of 10—the baby died. Now, the pharmacist went through her days with a distant glare to her eyes. She was talking of leaving the profession. The circumstance was tragic on multiple dimensions.

The hardest part of the job was coming to work and reviewing the list of babies for the day. RPG would inquire about baby so and so and be told she had gone to the seventh floor. It was the expression used by the staff to say the baby had died. The first year had not been too difficult. But now, RPG found she could not cope with her emotions regarding these babies, their circumstances, the impact on the parents' lives, and the increasing fear of making a fatal mistake. Sometimes, RPG found her hands shaking or her voice quivering as she worked through calculations or talked with the staff. Yesterday, she had gone home and yelled at her dog—she had never done that before. RPG found herself crying inappropriately at movies or while reading sentimental greeting cards. A dark gloom had settled over RPG's life that she couldn't shake. Talking with her friends, they noticed how she had changed in the past months. Her customary smile had turned to a lemony pucker of a frown. RPG was no longer having a good time at work.

How would you recommend RPG handle the situation?

Assignment: What Do the Practitioners/ Others Say?

BE PREPARED TO DISCUSS EMOTIONS based on any *one* of the following:

- A discussion with your colleagues, or others, on how they feel and what they know about emotions
- An article on emotions, either from the research literature or any other source
- A movie/television program/YouTube video about emotions
- A book on emotions (literary, historical, psychological, or any other source)

EXERCISES

The following exercises are intended to increase your mindfulness regarding your emotions. Mindfulness is the ability to be aware of your thoughts, emotions, physical sensations, and actions—in the present moment—without judging or criticizing yourself or your experience (McKay, Wood, & Brantley, 2007, p. 64). Mindfulness helps you gain a clearer understanding of your emotional world, the first step on the path to effectively managing your emotions.

Who Are My Emotional Role Models?

Our attitudes towards our emotions are derived from our earliest caregivers, typically family. Those we meet during childhood and adolescence shape our emotional world. Take a few moments to identify your emotional role models by answering the following questions:

Who were my emotional role models?_____

What was their emotional style? _____

What did I learn from them? _____

Source: Adapted from Spradlin, S. E. (2003). *Don't let your emotions run your life.* Oakland, CA: New Harbinger.

What Are My Emotional Triggers?

All of us have people and situations that provoke strong emotional reactions. Take a moment to consider what your emotional triggers are.

Describe a time you lost control of your emotions. _____

What was the precipitating event? _____

Is there a pattern to when you lose control of your emotions?

_____

What things cause you to lose your composure? _____

Describe Your Emotions

What does it feel like to be in love? _____

What does it feel like when you break up with someone? _____

What does it feel like when someone breaks up with you? _____

What were your feelings when your father came home from work? _____

What are your feelings when your boss comes in? _____

What were your feelings when you came for the interview for pharmacy school? _____

What emotions would you feel if you made a fatal medication error? _____

⊕ Emotional Catalogue

Use **Table 3.1** to keep a record of your emotions for a week, the events that caused them, their length, and their impact on the day.

TABLE 3.1   Emotional Catalogue

Date	Emotion	Circumstances (what happened, what was going on that day)
Monday		
Tuesday		
Wednesday		
Thursday		
Friday		
Saturday		
Sunday		

Based on this log, do you see any patterns? Are these patterns helpful, or not?

⫘ Temperament

Describe your predominant emotional temperament in one word.

_____

Check with family and friends to see if they agree.

⫘ Personal Learning Plan: Emotions

These steps can be compiled on a single page containing the following:

> What prompted me to develop this plan?
>
> What is the general area for improvement?
>
> What is the specific issue for improvement?
>
> Why is this important to me?
>
> How do I generally act in these areas?
>
> What are my goals?
>
> What prompted this effort?
>
> What strategies are required?
>
> Who/what is necessary to meet my goals with this strategy?
>
> How will I measure the success/failure of this effort?
>
> How long will I focus on this effort?
>
> How will I reflect and capture a lesson from this effort that can be generalized to other circumstances?

Based on your responses to the exercises, write a one-paragraph description of yourself as it relates to emotions.

⫘ WHAT'S IMPORTANT TO YOU IN THE CHAPTER?

With several of your classmates, discuss the idea/ideas that are most likely to effect a change in your values, attitudes, or behaviors. Be succinct—no more than two sentences.

⊪ REFERENCES

Goleman, D. (1995). *Emotional intelligence.* New York, NY: Bantam Dell.

McKay, M., Wood, J. C., & Brantley, J. (2007). *The dialectical behavior therapy skills workbook.* Oakland, CA: New Harbinger.

Segal, J. (1997). *Raising your emotional intelligence: A practical guide.* New York, NY: Owl.

Spradlin, S. E. (2003). *Don't let your emotions run your life.* Oakland, CA: New Harbinger.

⊪ SUGGESTED READINGS

Caruso, D. R., & Salovey, P. (2004). *The emotionally intelligent manager.* San Francisco, CA: Jossey-Bass.

Epstein, S. (1998). *Constructive thinking: The key to emotional intelligence.* Westport, CT: Praeger.

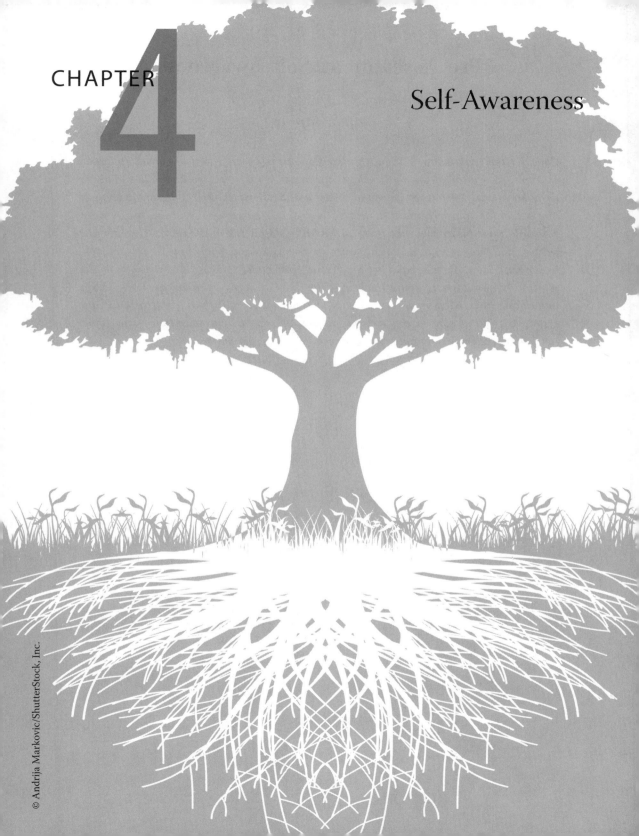

CHAPTER

4

Self-Awareness

Pre-Assessment: Self-Awareness

Mind Mapping

Consider the term below. Without thinking or editing, write down the ideas, concepts, examples, contradictions, and theories that come to mind. What words would you use to describe yourself? What words would others use to describe you? Do not array them in any systematic or orderly manner. Scatter them about the page. Now, draw lines between your additions indicating that there is a relationship between the terms. If something causes something else, indicate this with an arrow. Relationships may be reciprocal—both cause each other—requiring arrows at both ends. Indicate the strength of the relationship by darkening and thickening the lines; stronger relationships have darker and thicker lines. Most important: There is no right answer. Do not compare with your classmates. *What you have is a mind map, your mental representation of the topic. Review to determine if anything has changed following this chapter.*

Me

⪩ **DESIRED EDUCATIONAL OUTCOMES**

- Describe the concepts of self-awareness, self-observation, and self-insight.
- Describe why values are important.
- Define schemas.
- Define self-talk.

⪩ **DESIRED PERSONAL OUTCOME**

- Acquire enhanced personal awareness.

What Is Self-Observation?

SELF-OBSERVATION IS THE ACT OF paying attention to yourself—dispassionately, without criticism or evaluation. In a sense you become your own laboratory rat. Every aspect of your self is open to observation and scrutiny, including your core values, your emotions, your cognitive frames, the self-talk you engage in, your attitudes, your intentions, and more.

What Is Self-Awareness?

SELF-AWARENESS IS THE ABILITY TO focus on yourself as an object for observation and study. Self-awareness includes appraising yourself relative to a standard of conduct and reflecting on your behaviors in this broader context. If you have ever felt embarrassed after the fact for something you said or did, that is self-awareness.

Numerous thinkers have counseled that the formula for development, maturation, and success begins with an accurate picture of one's self and an understanding of how one behaves. Further, comparing yourself to a standard, either internal or external, and recognizing a gap in our ideal self and our actual self can be a catalyst for change.

What Is Self-Concept?

BY SELF-OBSERVING AND BECOMING SELF-AWARE, a self-concept emerges. The self-concept is relatively stable over time, consistent across situations, and not likely to change. It is your picture of yourself and is based on the internalized set of perceptions you have made regarding yourself. By these processes, you understand, as much as possible, your "modus operandi"— how you operate in the world. You come to understand why, for example, you thrive under pressure, or are reluctant to talk in class, or avoid conflict, the career choices you are considering, what things interest you, and on and on.

What Are the Barriers to Self-Awareness?

THERE ARE AT LEAST TWO barriers to acquiring an accurate picture of oneself. We all have a sensitive line regarding our self-awareness that we defend. In seeking to understand one's self, the individual acquires information that may be painful, or is inconsistent with their view of themselves. When this information challenges deeply held beliefs about our self and our self-worth, we tend to defend ourselves psychologically by offering explanations and rationales for this discrepancy. Information gained about ourselves that is verifiable relative to an objective standard, information about ourselves that is not unexpected, and information about ourselves over which we have some control as to content, quantity, and timing diminishes the discomfort associated with attacks on the sensitive line. In addition, information that is confirmed by others ameliorates the potential discomfort associated with the sensitive line. The implication of the sensitive line is that, when approached, we defend ourselves psychologically, thus limiting our chance for learning and further development.

The second barrier to self-understanding, particularly for pharmacy students, is time. Self-understanding requires conscious mental energy. It is work. What is gained is only what is put into it. One must take an active role as an observer. The crowded weekly calendar filled with classes, laboratories, study, clinical sites, work, extracurricular activities, and personal relationships simply doesn't leave the time or the psychic energy for most pharmacy students to indulge in the "luxury" of self-observation and self-awareness. Both self-observation and self-awareness require conscious mental activity. If none is available due to sheer exhaustion, then no insight will occur.

What Things Are Most Important to Learn About Myself?

T HERE ARE AN INFINITE NUMBER of things you could learn about yourself. Greater self-insight is an ongoing and lifelong activity. A good
starting point is to consider the following:

- What are my values?
- What schemas shape my understanding of the world?
- What self-talk do I engage in?

What Are Values?

Values are enduring and stable elements of our personality. They are the
constellation that sets the course of our life, impacts our decisions and
choices, reflects our tastes, and defines who we are. Values are not arrived
at rationally, but reflect our emotional world. Our values are anchored in
our country of origin, the specific culture within that country to which we
belong, and our families. It is important to note that individuals differ in
their level of value development. In other words, value priorities change
over a lifetime as people move through different stages of maturity. As individuals mature they tend to move from values related to the self through a
stage that focuses on conformity to external standards, and finally to a stage
that focuses on universal principles.

What Are Schemas?

A person's affect (feelings) and behaviors are based on the way they structure
the world. The verbal and pictorial events in our stream of consciousness
(cognitions) are derived from our basic attitudes and assumptions (schemas).
Schemas are pervasive themes that originate in childhood and are central to
your sense of self. If the schemas are maladaptive they translate into self-
defeating modes of operating. They are self-perpetuating. For example,
an individual abused as a child will tend to interpret all their experiences,
whether valid or not, from a framework of abuse. In short, how a person
thinks about the world determines how they feel and how they behave. A
schema is essentially your theory of how people and the world work.

What Is Self-Talk?

Self-talk is the inner monologue or dialogue that goes on in our brain. Self-talk is also referred to as "private speech" or "verbal rehearsal." Self-talk is used to solve problems, rehearse upcoming events, and challenge your assumptions about events. Self-talk helps you acquire information about yourself in that it increases private self-consciousness. If, after a conflict, you go over in your mind what you should have said, that is self-talk. Or if, after a poor golf shot, you tell yourself to forget it and go on with the next shot, that also is self-talk.

Self-Awareness at Work

THE FOLLOWING IS A SAMPLE scenario related to self-awareness involving RPG (recent pharmacy graduate):

RPG worked her way through pharmacy school with a "ne'er do well" husband strapped to her back. His goal, she found out as she got closer to graduating, was to semi-retire and hang out at the track with his buddies. As far as RPG was concerned this was not going to happen. The last year in school was a real hurdle—finishing the program, filing for a divorce, and studying for the boards. RPG still did not understand why she had married this guy.

Things were finally going well now, 2 years after graduation. RPG had her own house and a job she liked. Though the job was not perfect (she was slightly underpaid) it offered one real advantage: RPG wanted to get into consulting pharmacy and this job offered her the chance. Besides the usual pharmacist duties related to dispensing, RPG got to spend one day a week at the long-term care home reviewing charts. Once she became board certified in geriatrics, probably in a year, RPG would be on her way.

RPG had a terrible Christmas. Her father died in November and the holidays were strange without him. She felt disconnected. Thinking things over while she read the paper for a few moments before her shift started, RPG got a call from a recruiting firm. It was a management job in another long-term care facility. The recruiter said the job would involve directly managing one pharmacy and supervising a second facility about 50 miles away. The salary range was about $25,000 more than RPG was making now. The job was on the other side of town and would require a 75-minute commute. Overall, RPG really liked the work at her current job, but had some problems with some of the people she worked with.

RPG had no management experience, but the money was enticing. On the one hand the money excited RPG; on the other, when she began to consider the responsibility of managing these pharmacies, RPG was afraid.

How would you recommend RPG handle the situation?

Assignment: What Do the Practitioners/ Others Say?

BE PREPARED TO DISCUSS SELF-AWARENESS based on any *one* of the following:

• A discussion with your colleagues, or others, on the concept of self-awareness

• An article on self-awareness, either from the research literature or any other source

• A movie/television program/YouTube video about self-awareness

• A book on self-awareness (literary, historical, psychological, or any other source)

EXERCISES

What Are My Values?

As a pharmacy student, it is not likely that you have thought explicitly about your values. Most students are vaguely aware of what their values are. As should be expected, one's values will become clearer with experience. What follows is a brief exercise aimed at clarifying your values.

Answer the following questions:

As a student, what are the three most important things to me?

In my personal life, what are my three highest aspirations?

My career will be a success if I accomplish the following three things.

For each of the values listed, consider how much time you spend on a weekly basis in pursuit of these values.

Is Your Life Story

technique to aid in enhancing self-awareness is to take a few
:o write the story of your life. Divide a page into two columns.
r story on the left side of the page. On the right, note critical
l your reactions. Look for patterns and tendencies. Conclude the
a brief summary explaining these patterns and tendencies.

49

⊪ ɪ...ntifying My Self-Talk

Keep a pad and pencil by your bed. In the morning before you do anything
else, spend 15–20 minutes and write down whatever comes to mind. Do
not worry about style or editing. Capture all your thoughts whether complete or not. Do this for 3 weeks. Look for themes and patterns. Themes
and patterns of self-talk are reflective of the underlying schemas used to
understand the world.

Any afternoon, for 3 minutes record the thoughts and ideas that are
playing in your mind.

⊪ The Self-Talk Scale

Please answer using the following scale:
1 = never; 2 = seldom; 3 = sometimes; 4 = often; 5 = very often

I talk to myself when:

1. I should have done something differently (self-criticism) _____

2. Something good has happened to me (self-reinforcement) _____

3. I need to figure out what I should do or say (self-management) _____

4. I'm imagining how other people respond to things I've said (social
   assessment) _____

5. I am really happy for myself (self-reinforcement) _____

6. I want to analyze something that someone recently said to me (social
   assessment) _____

7. I feel ashamed of something I've done (self-criticism) _____

8. I'm proud of something I've done (self-reinforcement) _____

9. I'm mentally exploring a possible course of action (self-management) _____

10. I'm really upset with myself (self-criticism) _____

11. I try to anticipate what someone will say and how I'll respond to him or her (social assessment) _____

12. I'm giving myself instructions or directions about what I should do or say (self-management) _____

13. I want to reinforce myself for doing well (self-reinforcement) _____

14. Something bad has happened to me (self-criticism) _____

15. I want to remind myself of what I need to do (self-management) _____

16. I want to replay something that I've said to another person (social assessment) _____

Factors in parentheses indicate the focus of the self-talk.

Source: Brinthaupt, T. M., Hein, M. B., & Kramer, T. E. (2008). The self-talk scale: Development, factor analysis, and validation. *Journal of Personality Assessment, 91*(1), 92.

⫶⫶ Who Plays You in the Movies?

If your life were made into a movie, who would you cast to play you in the movie? Do not consider your idealized self, but the actor who most accurately represents you. See if your classmates agree.

⫶⫶ What Are My Schemas?

Review the list of schemas detailed here. See if any describe you. Most people will be combinations of schemas.

⫶⫶ Schemas

Not all schemas are negative. Most people resonate with one or more of these maladaptive schema. Maladaptive schema can be the source of many personal issues and problems. As such, they tend to provoke reflection and discussion. The goal is to convert maladaptive schema to functional schema.

Abandonment/Instability

Definition: The essence of this schema is the perceived instability or unreliability of those available for support and connection.

Origins: This schema develops when parents are extremely inconsistent in meeting the child's needs. Early experiences of loss, due to divorce, separation, illness, or death, are other obvious circumstances that lay the groundwork for the elaboration of this schema, as are the experiences of being always left alone or in the charge of numerous and constantly changing caretakers.

Characteristics: Because of their exaggerated fear of being left alone and abandoned, these people are usually very clingy in relationships, sometimes to the point of unwarranted jealousy.

Abuse/Mistrust

Definition: The essence of this schema involves the expectation that other people will hurt, abuse, humiliate, cheat, lie, manipulate, or take advantage of one. A fear of angry or violent outbursts from others is often included in the schema. People holding this schema experience other people's negative behaviors as intentional or as resulting from extreme and unjustifiable negligence.

Origins: This schema results from early childhood experiences of physical, sexual, or emotional abuse or from personal betrayal by parents or siblings.

Characteristics: Abused people are hypervigilant to harm, manipulation, or being cheated by others. They frequently distort events, read hidden meanings into statements, or attribute negative intentions to others' behavior. They can be accusatory, openly suspicious, and testing others' motives. If they think they are being cheated, they can behave in an unfeeling, cruel, or vengeful way.

Emotional Deprivation

Definition: Emotional deprivation involves the expectation that one's desire for a normal degree of emotional support will not be met by others. The person may feel deprived of nurturance, protection, or empathy. Deprivation of nurturance involves an absence of attention and warmth from others.

Origins: As already described, emotionally deprived people have usually experienced some form of emotional neglect during early childhood. Their parents are often cold, distant, nonempathic, weak, and unavailable. Consequently, these people expect that others will not be there to meet their needs.

Characteristics: Depending on the specific nature of the deprivation (nurturance, protection, or empathy), these people advertise their deprivation in both obvious and subtle ways. They can come across as demanding and controlling or can be cold, uncaring, insensitive, and withholding. Emotionally deprived people often report high levels of loneliness. Frequently, they avoid intimacy and closeness or pull away from nurturance because its unfamiliarity generates discomfort.

Functional Dependence/Incompetence

Definition: This schema relates to the feeling of not being able to handle one's everyday responsibilities competently or without considerable help from others.

Origins: This schema arises when parents do not encourage or allow a child to develop any sense of independence, competence, or self-sufficiency.

Characteristics: These people constantly avoid new tasks or even minor decisions; consequently, they present with a pervasive passivity. However, they attribute even real experiences of success or mastery to luck or a fluke.

Vulnerability to Harm and Illness

Definition: This schema involves an exaggerated fear that disaster—financial, medical, criminal, or natural—will strike at any time and that one is unable to protect oneself from disaster.

Origins: This schema usually results from having overly protective parents, who repeatedly conveyed the message, "The world is a dangerous place."

Characteristics: These people usually have a range of unrealistic fears—of having a heart attack, of getting AIDS, of going crazy or broke, of being mugged, and so on. They frequently suffer from anxiety disorders (panic disorder, generalized anxiety disorder, phobias, or hypochondriasis). The inherent unpredictability and uncertainty of everyday living is extremely anxiety-provoking to them.

Enmeshment/Undeveloped Self

Definition: The essence of this schema is excessive emotional closeness and involvement with one or more significant others at the expense of full individuation and normal social development.

Origins: This schema can arise within the context of a totally enmeshed family unit, in which the world is the family and everything outside is perceived as somehow less real or less meaningful. If the parents are extremely controlling, subjugating, or overprotective, the child may find it impossible to develop a separate sense of self.

Characteristics: Depending on their degree of enmeshment, these people find it extremely difficult to function separately from the family unit or enmeshing other. They spend a lot of time at home and usually remain living there well beyond the normal age for leaving the nest.

◀|▶ **Defectiveness/Shame**

Definition: This schema involves the feeling that one is inwardly defective, flawed, or invalid and that one is, therefore, fundamentally unlovable or unacceptable. Consequently, people who hold this schema have a deep sense of shame concerning their perceived internal inadequacies and a constant fear of exposure and further rejection by significant others.

Origins: This schema usually results from the experience of constant criticism, devaluation, or rejection by one or both parents. This behavior results in the conviction that one is inherently unacceptable and unlovable.

Characteristics: People holding this schema expect rejection and blame from others. They are therefore hypersensitive to even minor slights or criticisms. They are usually also very self-critical and exaggerate their own defects. By and large, they avoid intimacy and self-disclosure and therefore the risk of being exposed to rejection.

Social Undesirability/Alienation

Definition: This schema involves the belief that one is *outwardly* undesirable to, or different from, others. People may feel that they are ugly, sexually undesirable, poor in social skills, dull, boring, or low in status. Therefore, they feel self-conscious and insecure in social situations and have a sense of alienation or isolation from the rest of the world. These people frequently feel that they do not fit in, that they are not part of any group or community.

Origins: This schema can result from repeated criticism of certain aspects of appearance or social presentation. This is a familiar experience for children who grow up in an alcoholic household; they feel that their family has something to hide and is therefore less desirable than those of friends or peers.

Characteristics: These people feel more comfortable when alone because social situations trigger self-consciousness and perceived pressure to perform or to pretend that they are enjoying themselves. They usually minimize their social contacts or stay on the periphery of groups. Privately, they remain feeling totally detached and alienated.

Failure to Achieve

Definition: This schema involves the belief that one will inevitably fail or is fundamentally inadequate relative to one's peers in areas of achievement. It often involves the related belief that one is stupid, inept, untalented, or ignorant.

Origin: This schema often results from early criticism, usually by parents. Failure to achieve can also result from parents who are too demanding or set standards that are too high for the child; some children rebel against these excessive expectations by failing.

Characteristics: These people usually have a sense that they have failed in comparison to their peers, either at their job or at school. Often they actually are underachieving, but even people whose performance is adequate or excellent still have considerable anxiety concerning the possibility of failure.

Subjugation

Definition: This schema involves an excessive surrendering of control over one's own decisions and preferences—usually to avoid anger, retaliation, or abandonment.

Origins: This schema usually results from living with very controlling or domineering parents who punish, threaten to punish, or withdraw from the child for expressing his or her needs and wants. Sometimes parents simply override, and therefore negate, the child's wishes by enforcing their own.

Characteristics: Subjugated people frequently present a very compliant and unassertive picture. They exaggerate the likelihood of retribution if they express their needs rather than deferring to others. They are, therefore, excessively eager to please. Because they catastrophize the devastating impact of others' anger, they avoid conflict and confrontation at all costs. They frequently harbor anger at those they perceive as subjugating them, but their inability to manage and express this anger sometimes translates into passive-aggressive behavior.

Self-Sacrifice/Over-Responsibility

Definition: This schema involves a voluntary but excessive focus on meeting the needs of others at the expense of one's own gratification. The most common reasons for this self-sacrifice are to prevent causing pain to others, to maintain the connection with others who are perceived as more needy, to avoid guilt, or to gain in self-esteem. Self-sacrifice often results from an acutely tuned sensitivity to the pain of others. However, it leads to a feeling that one's own needs are not being met and sometimes to resentment of those for whom one sacrifices.

Origins: This schema can result from a child overidentifying with an emotionally needy parent and assuming the role of caretaker at an early age.

Characteristics: By and large, these people always put the needs of others first; in doing so, they tend to overextend and overcommit themselves. If they feel resentful that their needs are not being met by others, they may then feel guilty at their own selfishness. Guilt predominates—guilt that they caused the other person pain, guilt that they were not there when needed, guilt that they did not do the right thing, and guilt that they let the other person down. Guilt is the primary force in maintaining the schema.

Emotional Inhibition

Definition: This schema involves excessive inhibition of emotions and impulses—most frequently anger. The person expects the expression of emotions and impulses to result in loss of self-esteem, embarrassment, retaliation, abandonment, or harm to oneself or others.

Origins: Parents who discourage the expression of feelings, especially anger, and who either directly or tacitly convey that emotional control is a more acceptable and commendable aspiration than expression, lay the foundations for emotional inhibition.

Characteristics: Emotionally inhibited people can seem cold and controlled or logical and pragmatic to the point of lacking spontaneity and sensitivity. This is because they are very uncomfortable around displays of even positive emotions. They find it extremely difficult to handle their own emotions and frequently harbor fears of losing control. Socially, they are often construed as killjoys because their seriousness can make other people feel self-conscious and immature.

Unrelenting/Unbalanced Standards

Definition: This schema involves the relentless striving to meet high expectations of oneself at the expense of happiness, pleasure, relaxation, spontaneity, playfulness, health, and satisfying relationships.

Origins: Parents whose standards are very high and who deliver rewards such as love and attention contingent upon task completion or performance that meets high standards set the stage for unrelenting standards. Such parents often devalue the role of simple enjoyment and relaxation.

Characteristics: Predictably, these people are often very successful and accomplished, but they are also depressed and anxious or suffer from various psychosomatic complaints. They tend to exaggerate any deficits or flaws in themselves and to see things in rigid black-and-white categories. They work too hard, at the expense of feelings of well-being, good health, and relationships. In relationships, they look for perfection and can be very controlling and critical. In either case, these people tend not to invest the necessary time in their relationships; career pursuits and achievements take priority.

Entitlement/Self-Centeredness

Definition: Central to this schema is the feeling that one is entitled to whatever one wants—regardless of the cost to others or of what others or society might regard as reasonable.

Origins: These people have usually experienced extreme overindulgence and lack of responsibility as children.

Characteristics: People who hold this schema are egocentric and narcissistic. They have an exaggerated view of their own rights and worth in relation to others and the world and also an underdeveloped sense of their moral and social obligations. These people can, therefore, come across as arrogant, selfish, demanding, and controlling. They lack empathy for others' needs and tend to treat people carelessly. They often have an employment history of being fired because they could not get along with bosses or coworkers or of walking out when they did not get what they wanted.

Insufficient Self-Control/Self-Discipline

Definition: This schema involves pervasive difficulty exercising sufficient self-control or tolerating frustration long enough to achieve personal goals or to refrain from emotional outbursts or impulsive behaviors.

Origins: This schema can result from growing up in a household where limit setting was nonexistent or inconsistent, for example, where parents did not model self-control or adequately discipline the child or where one parent was very strict and the other very lax.

Characteristics: These people may exhibit problems of emotional and impulse control, overeating, alcohol and substance abuse, promiscuity, aggressive outbursts, and criminal behaviors.

Source: Adapted from Bricker, D., Young, J. E., & Flanagan, C. M. (1993). Schema-focused cognitive therapy: A comprehensive framework for characterological problems. In K. T. Kuehlwein & H. Rosen (Eds.), *Cognitive therapies in action* (pp. 92–113). San Francisco, CA: Jossey Bass.

⚡ Personal Learning Plan: Self-Awareness

These steps can be compiled on a single page containing the following:

> What prompted me to develop this plan?
>
> What is the general area for improvement?
>
> What is the specific issue for improvement?
>
> Why is this important to me?
>
> How do I generally act in these areas?
>
> What are my goals?
>
> What prompted this effort?
>
> What strategies are required?

Who/what is necessary to meet my goals with this strategy?

How will I measure the success/failure of this effort?

How long will I focus on this effort?

How will I reflect and capture a lesson from this effort that can be generalized to other circumstances.

Based on your responses to the exercises, write a one-paragraph description of yourself as it relates to self-awareness.

WHAT'S IMPORTANT TO YOU IN THE CHAPTER?

With several of your classmates, discuss the idea/ideas that are most likely to effect change in your values, attitudes, or behaviors. Be succinct—no more than two sentences.

REFERENCES

Bricker, D., Young, J. E., & Flanagan, C. M. (1993). Schema-focused cognitive therapy: A comprehensive framework for characterological problems. In K. T. Kuehlwein & H. Rosen (Eds.), *Cognitive therapies in action* (pp. 92–113). San Francisco, CA: Jossey Bass.

Brinthaupt, T. M., Hein, M. B., & Kramer, T. E. (2009). The self-talk scale: Development, factor analysis, and validation. *Journal of Personality Assessment, 91*(1), 82–92.

SUGGESTED READINGS

Beitman, B., Viamontes, G., Soth, A., & Nittler, J. (2006). Toward a neural circuitry of engagement, self-awareness, and pattern search. *Psychiatric Annals, 36*(4), 274–282.

Brach, T. (2003). *Radical acceptance.* New York, NY: Bantam.

DePape, A. R., Hakim-Larson, J., Voelker, S., Page, S., & Jackson, D. L. (2006). Self-talk and emotional intelligence in university students. *Canadian Journal of Behavioral Science, 38*(3), 250–260.

Kleiner, A., & Roth, B. (1997, September–October). How to make experience your company's best teacher. *Harvard Business Review*, 172–177.

Silvia, P., & Duval, T. S. (2001). Objective self-awareness theory: Recent progress and enduring problems. *Personality and Social Psychology Review*, 5(3), 230–241.

Sull, D. N., & Houlder, D. (2005, January). Do your commitments match your convictions? *Harvard Business Review*, 82–91.

Whetten, D., & Cameron, K. (2005). *Developing management skills* (6th ed.). Upper Saddle River, NJ: Pearson Education.

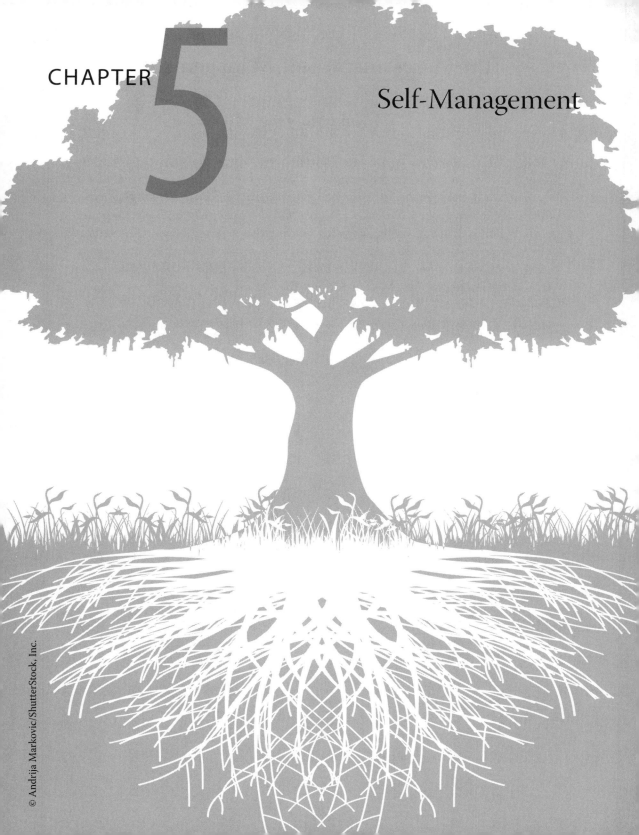

CHAPTER

5

Self-Management

Pre-Assessment: Self-Management

Mind Mapping

Consider the terms arrayed on the page. For each term, without thinking or editing, write down the ideas, concepts, examples, contradictions, and theories that come to mind. Do not array them in any systematic or orderly manner. Scatter them about the page. Now, draw lines between your additions, indicating that there is a relationship between the terms. If something causes something else, indicate this with an arrow. Relationships may be reciprocal—both cause each other—requiring arrows at both ends. Indicate the strength of the relationship by darkening and thickening the lines; stronger relationships have darker and thicker lines. Most important: There is no right answer. Do not compare with your classmates. *What you have is a mind map, your mental representation of the topic. Review to determine if anything has changed following this section.*

Self-control

Self-management

⊕ DESIRED EDUCATIONAL OUTCOME

- Describe strategies to regulate emotions.
- Discuss the ABC model and the impact of beliefs on behavior.

⊕ DESIRED PERSONAL OUTCOME

- Improve self-management.

What Are the Prerequisites for Self-Management?

THE FIRST STEP IN SELF-MANAGEMENT is eliminating psychological dissonance in your life. Whenever possible, the things you have to do should be aligned with the things you like to do. If work is a constant irritant and doesn't meet your inner psychic needs, then you will always be out of sorts. Your emotions will always be close to the surface. Consider how abrupt you might be with someone if you had suffered from a toothache all day. Psychic pain caused by a lack of congruence in your life will have the same effect. Imagine life as a community pharmacist if you always wanted to work in a hospital.

The second step in self-management is summed up in this quote by M. Scott Peck (2003, p. 15): "Life is difficult This is the great truth, one of the greatest truths—it is a great truth because once we see this truth, we transcend it." Think over your life. Has there ever been a day when you weren't worried about something, afraid of something, apprehensive about something? Small children, less than 5 years old, go off to preschool concerned that one of their friends didn't play with them yesterday. To be alive is to have problems and worries. Understanding this, it is easier to keep things in perspective. Although life may go up and down, your perspective on events and your response to those peaks and valleys can smooth out their emotional impact. Remember, the only time all your wants and needs were completely satisfied was in the womb.

What Is at the Core of Self-Management?

A NATIVE AMERICAN CHIEF IS TALKING to his tribe about two dogs inside his mind: one a white dog that is good and courageous, the other a black dog that is vengeful and angry. A young brave, unable to wait for the end of the story, asks, "Which one will win?" the chief responds, "The one I feed." The ultimate key to self-management is to recognize that you are in control of everything you feel, everything you think, and how you behave. No other person—*no one*—makes you feel or think or do anything. Dr. Seuss in *Oh, the Places You'll Go!* summed this point as well as anyone: "You have brains in your head. You have feet in your shoes. You can steer yourself any direction you choose. You're on your own and you know what you know. And YOU are the guy who'll decide where to go."

What Is Emotional Regulation and Self-Management?

EMOTIONAL REGULATION IS THE PROCESS by which individuals modulate their emotions. The goal is to control the intensity, duration, occurrence, or expression of emotions. Self-management does not mean that one never feels emotions, or never lets them show. It would be a cold heart that rounded on a pediatric floor with children suffering from leukemia and felt nothing. Denial of emotions is not the ideal. Nor is the universal suppression of emotions the ideal. A child who violates a mutually agreed-upon course of action should see and experience a measure of a parent's displeasure. In talking to a patient about a life-threatening circumstance, they should sense your caring and concern. But, if you face a crisis situation in a neonatal intensive care unit, it is necessary to suppress your anxiety so that you can function most effectively. In other words, feeling emotion is fine, showing emotion is fine, and suppressing emotion is fine. A self-managed individual knows which response is appropriate for any circumstance and can execute the appropriate response. This is a difficult admonition. These situations are subtle, fluid, and multilayered. An expectation that one can be perfect at this is unreasonable. The standard by which to measure oneself on this pursuit is improvement, not perfection.

In his book *Tuesdays with Morrie* (2002), Mitch Albom captures the idea of emotional management and self-regulation.

> If you hold back on your emotions—if you don't allow yourself to go all the way through them—you can never get back to being detached, you're too busy being afraid. You're afraid of the pain, you're afraid of the grief. You're afraid of the vulnerability that love entails. But by throwing yourself into those emotions, by allowing yourself to dive in, all the way, over your head even, you experience them fully and completely. You know what pain is, you know what love is. You know what grief is. And only then can you say, "All right." I have experienced that emotion. I recognize that emotion. Now I need to detach from that emotion for a moment. (p. 104)

What Are Specific Strategies for Emotional Regulation?

I N MANAGING YOUR EMOTIONS AND managing yourself, the following options are available:

- Don't put yourself in situations that you know have the potential to cause you to lose control or focus. Recall what your hot buttons are. What are the people, places, and circumstances that over time have caused you to lose your composure? Just stay away from them.

- If you can, alter situations that have the potential for causing you to lose control. If a specific individual gets under your skin, try never to meet with them alone. The presence of others may moderate your reaction to them.

- Focus on those aspects of people and circumstances that do not arouse you rather than the elements that do.

- Reappraise the circumstances that cause emotional turmoil. When taking a critical test, realizing that it is just a series of questions on a piece of paper rather than a measure of your self-worth blunts its emotional power.

- Control and modulate your response to the arousing circumstances. In other words, take a deep breath or walk away for a moment, alter your thought process, and respond rather than react unthinkingly. At the extreme, the emotion is suppressed. If your residency director has a bad day and takes it out on you, it is probably a good idea to quietly take it, rather than lashing back.

The one response that is always in your control is your ability to reappraise circumstances, to frame things in such a way that your emotional response is appropriate.

What Is Cognitive Reappraisal and Self-Management?

"THE GOAL OF EFFECTIVE LIVING is to think effectively: to know when we have crazy ideas" (Friday, 1999, p. 15). This idea captures the essence of effective self-management—that is, to think appropriately about the circumstances of your life. Cognitive reappraisal and self-management mean that you manage and control your thoughts. If something happens to you, an angry customer for example, that experience can be termed an activating event. Because of that event you respond in a certain way; for example, you lash back at the customer. That is the consequence of the event. What is missing from this scenario, and that determines your response both emotionally and behaviorally, is the belief about the event. If you believe the customer is a rude, demeaning individual then you might feel justified in lashing out at the person. If you believe the customer is a human being worthy of respect and consideration, no matter their behavior, or that the patient has significant health concerns, then you are likely to behave with professionalism, compassion, and empathy. This sequence can be reduced to the easily understood formula:

$$A \text{ (activating event)} + B \text{ (belief)} = C \text{ (consequence)}$$

Effective thinking means that you examine the beliefs you apply to any circumstance to see if they meet an empirical test (Where is the proof that this belief is true?), a functional test (Does my belief help me or make things worse?), and a logical test (Does it meet a test for common sense?). Self-management requires that you engage in an internal debate with yourself, that you dispute with yourself the validity of your beliefs. If your beliefs are found wanting, then your task is to alter them so that your beliefs, and hence your behaviors, are functional.

Let me emphasize, control of your belief in any situation is the basis of self-management. As Gandhi observed:

> Your beliefs become your thoughts.
>
> Your thoughts become your words.
>
> Your words become your actions.
>
> Your actions become your habits.
>
> Your habits become your values.
>
> Your values become your destiny.

Your self-managed destiny begins when you accept that you are in control of your emotions and thoughts.

Self-Management at Work

THE FOLLOWING IS A SAMPLE scenario related to self-management involving RPG (recent pharmacy graduate):

> It had been a long and tedious winter. Now spring was just around the corner. RPG could start to sense the shift in the weather. For some reason this winter had impacted RPG more than normal. RPG found it difficult every day to get up and adopt a positive attitude. In the back of his mind, RPG knew that his elderly father did not look good the last time he saw him. He knew that within a short time he would have to confront the issue of his father's demise. Also, RPG didn't know what it was, but his long-time personal relationship was tense. The two of them could not seem to connect with one another. What, at one time, had seemed easy now was a struggle. Bundled together, these factors left RPG with a base feeling of discontent.

How would you recommend RPG handle the situation?

Assignment: What Do the Practitioners/ Others Say?

B E PREPARED TO DISCUSS SELF-MANAGEMENT based on any *one* of the following:

- A discussion with your colleagues, or others, on the concept of self-management
- An article on self-management, either from the research literature or any other source
- A movie/television program/YouTube video about self-management
- A book on self-management (literary, historical, psychological, or any other source)

 EXERCISES

⚓ Perspective

Describe the biggest emotional crisis of your high school years. How important is this event to you now?

Describe the biggest emotional event of your college career. How important is it to you now?

Write down your grade point average and class standing. How important do you think these will be in 20 years?

If you were given a terminal diagnosis today, what event in your past life would still be important today?

⚓ Fake It

One way to deal with and control your emotions is to act the opposite of how you feel. In a sense, you are going to "fake it until you make it."

Anger: If you are feeling angry, what behaviors that are the opposite of anger could you engage in to moderate your responses? _____

Fear: If you are feeling afraid, what behaviors that are the opposite of fear could you engage in to moderate your responses? _____

Sadness: If you are felling sad, what behaviors that are the opposite of sad could you engage in to moderate your responses? _____

If confronted with a situation that you know will cause you to lose control, consider the following:

Think of a similar situation that you handled well and re-create it in your mind. Now transpose to the current situation and visualize a successful conclusion. _____

If you have never handled such a situation, or never handled it well, think of someone you know who would be good at this. Visualize how they would handle it. _____

If you don't have an acquaintance that comes to mind, think of a movie character that would be good in this situation. Visualize how he or she would handle it. _____

⫷ Examine Your Beliefs

1. With several classmates, discuss and isolate the collective belief about performance on a test.

2. With several classmates, discuss and isolate the collective belief about talking in class.

Do these beliefs meet the test for effective thinking? Specifically, do they meet an empirical test (Where is the proof that this belief is true?), a functional test (Does my belief help me or make things worse?), or a logical test (Does it meet a test for common sense?).

⫷ Personal Learning Plan: Self-Management

These steps can be compiled on a single page containing the following:

What prompted me to develop this plan?

What is the general area for improvement?

What is the specific issue for improvement?

Why is this important to me?

How do I generally act in these areas?

What are my goals?

What prompted this effort?

What strategies are required?

Who/what is necessary to meet my goals with this strategy?

How will I measure the success/failure of this effort?

How long will I focus on this effort?

How will I reflect and capture a lesson from this effort that can be generalized to other circumstances?

Based on your responses to the exercises, write a one-paragraph description of yourself as it relates to self-management.

⊕ WHAT'S IMPORTANT TO YOU IN THE CHAPTER?

With several of your classmates, discuss the idea/ideas that are most likely to effect a change in your values, attitudes, or behaviors. Be succinct—no more than two sentences.

⊕ REFERENCES

Albom, M. (2002). *Tuesdays with Morrie*, New York, NY: Broadway Books.
Friday, P. J. (1999). *Friday's laws.* Pittsburgh, PA: Bradley Oak.
Peck, M. S. (2003). *The road less traveled.* New York, NY: Simon and Schuster.

⊕ SUGGESTED READINGS

Chodron, P. (2002). *The places that scare you.* Boston, MA: Shambhala.
Ellis, A. (2001). *New directions for rational emotive therapy.* Amherst, NY: Prometheus.

Epstein, S. (1998). *Constructive thinking*. Westport, CT: Praeger.

Glasser, W. (1985). *Positive addiction*. New York, NY: Harper and Rowe.

Gross, J. J., & Thompson, R. A. (2007). Emotion regulation. In J. J. Gross (Ed.), *Handbook of emotion regulation* (pp. 3–24). New York, NY: Guilford Press.

McKay, M., Wood, J. C., & Brantley, J. (2007). *The dialectical behavior therapy skills workbook*. Oakland, CA: New Harbinger.

Orloff, J. (2009). *Emotional freedom*. New York, NY: Harmony.

Paprikh, J. *Managing your self*. (1991). Malden, MA: Blackwell Publishing.

Schutte, N. S., Manes, R. R., & Malouff, J. M. (2009). Antecedent-focused emotion regulation, response modulation and well-being. *Current Psychology, 28*, 21–31.

Spradlin, S. E. (2003). *Don't let your emotions run your life*. Oakland CA: New Harbinger.

Szasz, P. L., Szentagotai, A., & Hofmann, S. G. (2001). The effect of emotion regulation strategies on anger. *Behavior Research and Therapy, 49*, 114–119.

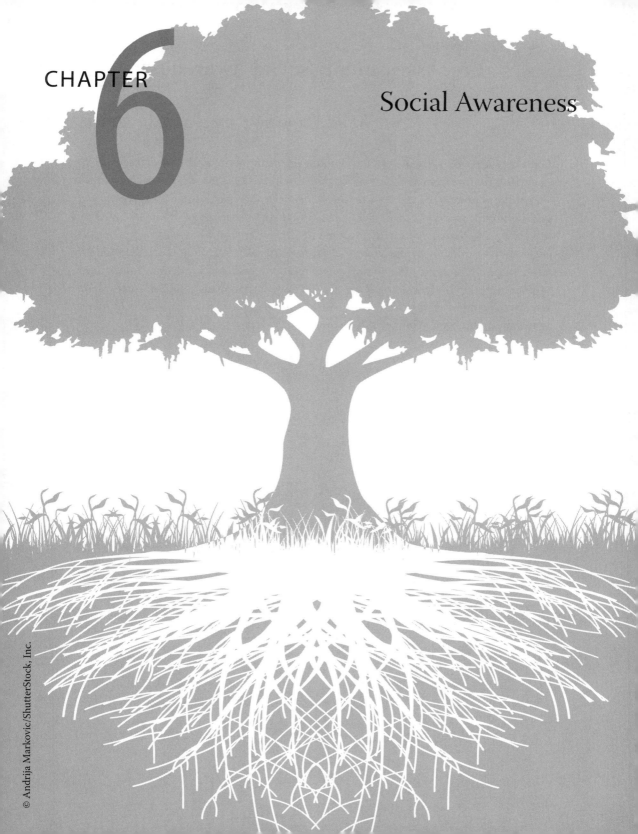

CHAPTER

6

Social Awareness

Pre-Assessment: Social Awareness

Mind Mapping

Consider the phrases below. Without thinking or editing, write down the ideas, concepts, examples, contradictions, and theories that come to mind. Do not array them in any systematic or orderly manner. Scatter them about the page. Now, draw lines between your additions indicating that there is a relationship between the terms. If something causes something else, indicate this with an arrow. Relationships may be reciprocal—both cause each other—requiring arrows at both ends. Indicate the strength of the relationship by darkening and thickening the lines; stronger relationships have darker and thicker lines. Most important: There is no right answer. Do not compare with your classmates. What you have is a mind map, your mental representation of the topic. Review to determine if anything has changed following this section.

Reading people
Who is a friend
Who is telling the truth

⬥ DESIRED EDUCATIONAL OUTCOMES

- Discuss the concept of social awareness.
- Discuss the impact of emotional blinders.
- Discuss intuition and social awareness.
- Describe how to improve social awareness.

⬥ DESIRED PERSONAL OUTCOME

- Enhance social awareness.

What Is Social Awareness?

IN A COMMUNITY SETTING, ALL pharmacists need to acquire the ability to quickly and accurately assess everyone walking into the pharmacy. First, are they a problem? Are they here for legitimate reasons, or might they hurt me? Are they really sick? Do they need special considerations for their circumstances? Did they just come from the doctor with a life-threatening diagnosis? Have they just been dismissed from the emergency room—can you see the pain in their face? Do I believe they will be compliant and follow both the doctor's orders and my counseling? Can they understand what I am explaining to them? The list of required observations for a pharmacist is exhaustive. Further, the art of being a first-rate clinician is grounded in the ability to glean information about patients and their condition not only from their chart, but also from their presentation, their mannerisms, their speech—from everything about them. Accurately reading each and every case is an exercise in the art of social awareness; it is the ability to sense the environment and act accordingly.

Pharmacists in today's world seldom work alone. Interaction with other pharmacists, techs, physicians, nurses, patient families, and administrators is at the center of today's practice environment. It is the essence of being part of the healthcare team. Is this a pharmacist who performs well under pressure, or does he or she become anxious? Is the tech a bit slow today due to a late night, or something more troubling? Is this a doctor I can approach? Which nurse is the one I should go to when I have a problem on the floor? Which nurse is the one to avoid because she has never liked the pharmacy department? Is this a patient's family I can work with, or will they be difficult? Which administrators may be trying to cut the pharmacy budget, and which administrator is an advocate for the pharmacy department? Successfully negotiating winning responses to situations such as these requires the ability to read situations and read people—in short, to be socially aware and mindful of what is happening around you.

What Are Emotional Blinders?

IRONICALLY, GIVEN THAT EMOTIONAL INTELLIGENCE is the focus of this work, excessive emotions cloud our judgment by blinding us to social cues in the environment. If you are romantically interested in someone you often miss the cues they send you. For example, if you are surprised by a break-up, many of your friends (relatively disinterested and emotionally neutral) will say they could see it coming. If, as a graduating pharmacy student, you desperately want to move to a certain part of the country to practice, you may neglect or minimize troubling aspects related to the quality of the work environment. Or, if the pharmacist in charge has upset you, you may miss obvious cues regarding certain patients. In short, at the extreme your emotions may blind you to your social environment.

Other states of mind also contribute to missing cues when regarding people. The first is neediness, which is characterized by the axiom "Never shop when you are hungry." If you need something more than you would normally, or you want something more than another person, then your ability to read people and circumstances is suspect. The second is fear. If, for example, you are fearful of being alone you may not notice troubling patterns in the behavior of someone you have a relationship with. The third state of mind that will inhibit the ability to read people is defensiveness. Once you are engaged in defending your ego against attack or uncomfortable information, you are not likely to notice relevant cues in your environment.

What Is Intuition?

WITH APPROPRIATE EMOTIONAL CONTROL YOU can exercise a powerful psychological mechanism for making sense of your world—intuition. Intuition occurs outside of conscious thought. It is a holistic and

integrating associative process. Finely tuned intuition allows you to see patterns in ill-defined and sloppy situations. It is the subconscious application
of previous learning to a current situation. Intuition can be characterized
as automated expertise. Having seen thousands of patients, intuition allows
you to look at a patient with a new prescription and know that something
is wrong without exactly knowing why or how you made this determination. Intuition is at work when you say this situation "feels OK," or "I have
a funny feeling in the pit of my stomach." A pharmacy student might have a
job offer that meets all their criteria for acceptance—hours, salary, working
conditions, and so on; however, when visiting the pharmacy something just
doesn't feel right. Intuition is a powerful mechanism in reading social cues.
Not honoring it is often a prelude to problems.

How Can I Improve My Social Awareness?

JURY CONSULTANTS SPECIALIZE IN READING people and circumstances
related to the selection of potential jurors for trials. People's lives and mil-
lions of dollars often hang on their recommendations. What follows are
brief points from this arena that are aimed at improving social awareness:

- *Scan:* At any one time an overload of information is available for
  attention and processing. To deal with this issue, first scan the situation. What is the backdrop, the physical aspects of the situation, the
  room, the people? In other words, try to see the big picture. While
  doing this, search for subtle clues that might be telling.

- *Pare:* Next, pare this information down to the aspects that stand out.
  What catches your eye, your ear, your other senses? What aspects of
  this situation pertain directly to the task at hand?

- *Enlarge:* Having identified the specific aspects of the situation most
  relevant to you, bring these features into sharper focus. Concentrate
  on these aspects.

- *Evaluate:* Having focused on and enlarged specific aspects, now
  evaluate them. Do you see patterns? Are there deviations from normal behaviors? Look for extremes.

- *Decide:* Make a decision based on this process. If possible, test whether your hypothesis is correct. Finally, practice this process as you seek to improve your abilities to read people and situations.

Being socially aware is no different than being an effective clinician. The task is the same, only the context varies. In both cases the task is to see both the trees and the forest. If you call a pediatrician with a sick child, their questions center on specific markers: what is the baby's temperature, is there a discharge from the nose, a cough, and so on. Ultimately, they will ask the mother whether the baby looks sick. In other words, they want specific markers from the mother and a global assessment of the baby's condition.

What's the Critical Element in Reading People?

IN THE SOCIAL CONTEXT YOU read vast amounts of information. You either explicitly attend to or unconsciously absorb this information. You run mental checklists or intuitively draw conclusions. You analyze the "shows" that people want you to understand about them and their unconscious "tells" that give them away. You process your first and subsequent impressions of people. You will never be completely right in reading someone. What you can do is gather enough information to establish a consistent pattern. If pieces of information about people present an incongruent picture, then you should be cautious. If you have an assessment of someone or a situation that seems to hang together or make sense, then this is probably the best you can do.

In developing a consistent, patterned picture of someone's character or emotions the following points are useful:

- *Get a first impression.* Form a first impression based on a person's most striking trait. As you acquire more information, confirm or disconfirm your first impressions.

- *What's unusual?* Extremes and deviations from patterns are important.

- *Is it temporary or permanent?* People vary on a daily basis; they are up and down. Is what you are seeing a trend or a single aberrant event?

- *Is what you are seeing due to choice or fate?* We can all choose to present in many different ways, depending on our needs and circumstances. Nonelective traits have a more pervasive impact on our emotions and behaviors. An extremely small person can choose to dress stylishly and meticulously, but can never escape the shaping influence of stature.

- *Some traits are more revealing.* An individual's level of compassion, socioeconomic background, and contentment with life often reveal more about an individual than do other traits.

Social Awareness at Work

THE FOLLOWING IS A SAMPLE scenario related to social awareness involving RPG (recent pharmacy graduate):

RPG reviewed the prescriptions for a new patient. The prescriptions called for what appeared to be excessive doses of muscle relaxers and amphetamine. RPG had judiciously worked to make sure that patients did not view her pharmacy as one that would fill any prescriptions with no questions asked. This approach was taken to limit the word of mouth on the street and thus eliminate questionable patients from her clientele. If RPG sensed the prescriptions were questionable, but probably legal, she told the patients she would have to order the drugs and it would take several days. Such patients then generally asked for their prescriptions back and left.

RPG glanced at the prescriptions and the patient in front of her. Nothing was alarming about the patient's appearance. Patients with questionable prescriptions presented either with a practiced air of nonchalance or a fidgety concern. This patient had a look of concern on her face, but it was different.

How would you recommend RPG handle the situation?

Assignment: What Do the Practitioners/ Others Say?

BE PREPARED TO DISCUSS SOCIAL awareness based on any *one* of the following:

- A discussion with your colleagues, or others, on the concept of social awareness
- An article on social awareness, either from the research literature or any other source
- A movie/television program/YouTube video about social awareness
- A book on social awareness (literary, historical, psychological, or any other source)

 EXERCISES

⊪ Who Is a Millionaire?

As an exercise in social awareness, go to any location and try to pick out who is the millionaire, or who has the most money.

What are the markers for this? _____

How might they be confusing? _____

⊪ What's Really Going On?

Watch a movie with the sound off. Can you determine what is happening in the scene?

⊪ Who Is Romantically Interested?

How do you tell if someone is romantically interested in you?

What are the specific markers for this?

If he or she were from a different culture would it be more complicated? Why?

〰 How Do Men and Women Look at Each Other?

If a man sees an attractive woman on the street, what does he do? What is his reaction?

If a woman sees an attractive man on the street, what does she do? What is her reaction?

〰 Who Is a Problem Patient?

How do you tell if a patient is going to be a problem?

〰 Explain the Haircut

Take a few moments and speculate on what the hairstyles shown in **Figures 6.1** and **6.2** say about these people.

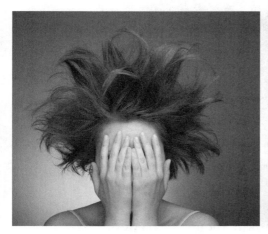

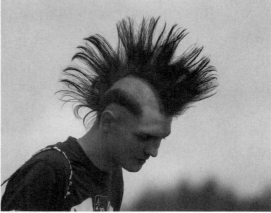

Figure 6.1   Hairstyle 1.
(Image © Jessmine/ShutterStock, Inc.)

Figure 6.2   Hairstyle 2.
(Image © Iakov Filimonov/ShutterStock, Inc.)

⚹ Write a Story

Write a one-paragraph story explaining what is going on with the woman in **Figure 6.3**. Compare your version to others in the class.

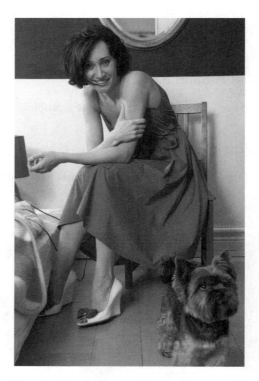

Figure 6.3   What is going on with this woman?
(Image © Elena Rostunova/ShutterStock, Inc.)

⚹ Personal Learning Plan: Social Awareness

These steps can be compiled on a single page containing the following:

What prompted me to develop this plan?

What is the general area for improvement?

What is the specific issue for improvement?

Why is this important to me?

How do I generally act in these areas?

What are my goals?

What prompted this effort?

What strategies are required?

Who/what is necessary to meet my goals with this strategy?

How will I measure the success/failure of this effort?

How long will I focus on this effort?

How will I reflect and capture a lesson from this effort that can be general-ized to other circumstances?

Based on your responses to the exercises, write a one-paragraph description of yourself as it relates to social awareness.

WHAT'S IMPORTANT TO YOU IN THE CHAPTER?

With several of your classmates, discuss the idea/ideas that are most likely to effect change in your values, attitudes, or behaviors. Be succinct—no more than two sentences.

SUGGESTED READINGS

Bradberry, T., & Greaves, J. (2005). *The emotional intelligence quickbook*. New York, NY: Fireside.

Dimitrius, J. E., & Mazzarella, W. P. (2008). *Reading people*. New York, NY: Ballantine.

Hayashi, A. M. (2001, February). When to trust your gut. *Harvard Business Review*, 59–65.

Hodgkinson, G. P., Langan-Fow, J., & Sadler-Smith, E. (2008). Intuition: A fundamental bridging construct in the behavioral sciences. *British Journal of Psychology, 99*, 1–27.

Kasar, J., & Clark, E. N. (2000). *Developing professional behaviors*. Thorofare, NJ: Slack.

McKenna, J. A. (2005). *Beyond tells: Power poker psychology*. New York, NY: Kensington.

Orlogg, J. (2009). *Emotional freedom*. New York, NY: Harmony.

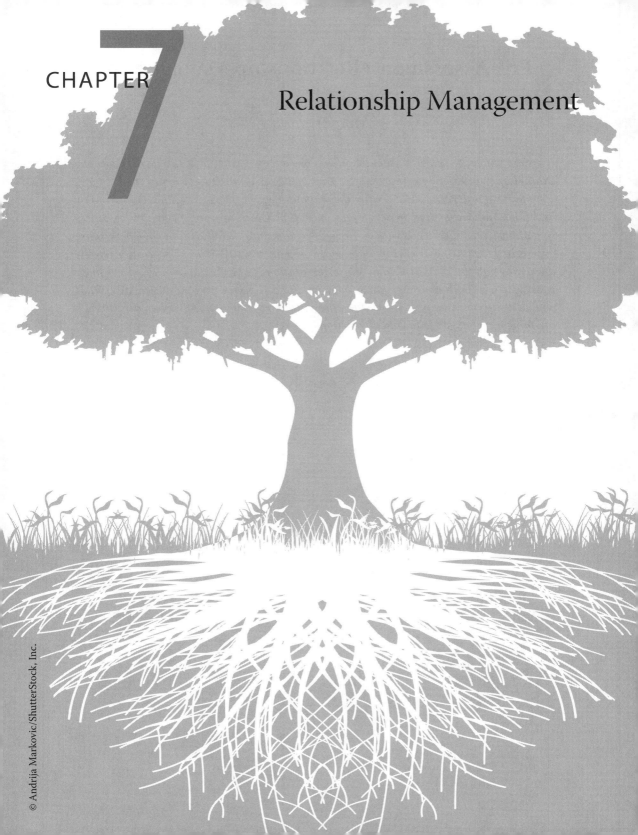

7

Relationship Management

Pre-Assessment: Relationship Management

Mind Mapping

Consider the term below. Without thinking or editing, write down the ideas, concepts, examples, contradictions, and theories that come to mind. Do not array them in any systematic or orderly manner. Scatter them about the page. Now, draw lines between your additions, indicating that there is a relationship between the terms. If something causes something else, indicate this with an arrow. Relationships may be reciprocal—both cause each other—requiring arrows at both ends. Indicate the strength of the relationship by darkening and thickening the lines—stronger relationships have darker and thicker lines. Most important: There is no right answer. Do not compare with your classmates. *What you have is a mind map, your mental representation of the topic. Review to determine if anything has changed following this section.*

Relationships

⫸ DESIRED EDUCATIONAL OUTCOMES

- Describe the concept of transference.
- List your rights in a relationship.
- Describe a toxic relationship.
- Describe what characterizes a successful relationship.

⫸ DESIRED PERSONAL OUTCOME

- Improved relationship skills.

What Is the Neurobiology of Relationships?

A CELTIC PROVERB SAYS THAT "we live in the shadow of each other." All humans are inherently social animals. In a famous experiment, psychologist Harry Harlow demonstrated that an infant rhesus monkey preferred the comfort of a warm, cloth-covered surrogate mother to one that dispensed nutrition. The developing human brain is constructed via interactions the individual has with other humans. In short, who we are is a function of the human relationships that have shaped us. Without stimulating relationships human beings wither and die. Human connections create tangible neuronal connections. Hebb's law declares that "Neurons that fire together wire together." From an evolutionary perspective, our neural circuitry is wired for both self-protection and social connection. A significant part of our neural circuitry is wired for reading social cues. Connecting into groups and maintaining relationships is a mechanism for human survival.

Recently, mirror neurons were discovered in the human brain. When mirror neurons fire they allow one human being to mimic, or mirror, what another human being does. Mirror neurons allow one human to create the mental state of another inside him- or herself. Because of mirror neurons we can get an immediate, visceral sense of another human being, letting us experience points of connection, empathy, and resonance.

The Relationship Is Good, So Why Is It So Hard Sometimes?

RELATIONSHIPS ARE WORK. Successful relationships don't just happen. Everyone has a myriad of needs, wants, and aspirations, some of which they are not even aware of. Inevitably, frictions result as two people pursue these needs, wants, and aspirations. A good counsel to keep in mind is that other people are not out to take advantage of you; but they are out for themselves. Some days the easiest thing would be to just say what you think and feel without any regard to the consequences. Some days the easiest thing would be to just end the relationship. A successful relationship is one where the fundamentals are good—at the core both people resonate with one another and both are willing to do the work to sustain the relationship. The key point is that just because a relationship takes work does not mean that it is defective.

If I'm in a Relationship, Shouldn't I Be Selfless?

ON THE SMALL THINGS—WHAT to have for dinner, what color to paint the room—a willingness to accommodate is the lubricant that makes relationships work. But on the core issues, like how many children to have, attitudes towards money, and career aspirations, the admonition is that it is OK to be selfish. Trading away your dreams for a relationship will only beget anger, resentment, and hostility. If the individuals are mature they will work out their differences; if not, these felt resentments will emerge surreptitiously. Ultimately, these issues will need to be addressed or the relationship will end, either formally or by becoming a hollow shell populated by two cynical and disinterested parties.

If They Would Only . . .

A FAMILIAR REFRAIN IN DEALING WITH another person is something like, "Things would be OK if you would just. . . ." Implicit in this comment is the notion that the relationship would improve if the other person would change. And if they won't change, my task is to change them to suit my needs. This misses the key point regarding change in humans: you can never change another person. If the relationship is difficult and in trouble, the only aspect you control is yourself. If you change, then the other person will change. Reciprocity accounts for this phenomenon. Want someone to be more considerate of your feelings? Then be considerate of theirs. Want someone to be more open about their issues? Then be open about your issues. As indicated at the beginning of this chapter, there is biological support for this point in that we all possess mirror neurons designed such that we mimic one another. You are only responsible for you; you are not responsible for the other person's behavior.

What Is Reciprocity?

THE ESSENCE OF ANY RELATIONSHIP is two people trying to get what they want. People in a relationship can be conceptualized as being in a dance together that they collectively choreograph via their actions and reciprocal reactions toward one another. A well-choreographed dance results in an upward spiraling relationship based on active listening, communication, empathy, negotiation, and problem solving. A poor relationship results in a downward spiral characterized by the opposite dimensions of the previous sentence. Successful relationships are based on a psychological contract of supportive reciprocity; in other words, I will get from you the things I provide you.

What Are My Rights in the Relationship?

RELATIONSHIPS REQUIRE MINDFUL ATTENTION. To maintain and strengthen relationships we must assert ourselves in an appropriate manner. Passive acceptance and disregard are not the path to a functioning relationship. In asserting ourselves regarding the relationship, it is permissible to ask for what you want, it is OK to say no, and you must negotiate conflict without damaging the relationship. In strengthening and maintaining relationships it is helpful to understand the "rights" that both of you have in the relationship. Those rights are (adapted from McKay, Wood, & Brantley, 2007):

- To need things
- To be first sometimes
- To ask for help
- To say no
- To sometimes inconvenience or disappoint

What Is Transference?

A KEY POINT REGARDING RELATIONSHIPS is the understanding that no relationship is new. All current relationships are colored by previous relationships. The term for this phenomenon is *transference*, and it occurs at an unconscious level. Humans' most potent relationships are with their earliest caregivers. These early relationships are internalized and idealized. The first "organization" for all of us is the family. It is the notion of transference that explains why having had an autocratic father who was overbearing, we now find ourselves inexplicably arguing with our male boss. We unconsciously act as if our boss was our father. If you have ever taken an instant dislike to someone, for no apparent reason other than the way he or she looks and acts, transference is the likely explanation.

What Is a Toxic Relationship?

S OMETIMES PEOPLE FIND THEMSELVES IN a toxic relationship, one where you are asked to sacrifice all of your needs for the enrichment of the other. Such relationships are best exemplified by cult leaders. In personal relationships, extreme infatuation with another person leads an individual to sacrifice everything to maintain the relationship. There is a sense of complete fulfillment. No other human can completely fulfill your needs. Insecurity and the need to feel special drive such a relationship. Needless to say, toxic relationships don't turn out well for one of the parties. The best that can be said of toxic relationships is to avoid them.

What Characterizes a Successful Relationship?

LONG-TERM, SUCCESSFUL RELATIONSHIPS ARE CHARACTERIZED by the following (adapted from Tamm & Luyet, 2004):

- *Collaborative intent:* Partners in a relationship make a mutual commitment to the relationship.

- *Truthfulness:* Partners commit to both telling and listening to the truth. This is accomplished by creating an atmosphere of openness and trust where the difficult issues can be considered.

- *Self-accountability:* Partners accept responsibility for their lives, the choices they make, and the consequences of their choices. Accountability trumps blaming.

- *Awareness of self and others:* Partners in the relationship commit to enhancing self-awareness, and understanding the context of their circumstances and the issues that motivate others.

- *Problem solving:* Partners in the relationship commit to engaging in effective problem solving rather than subtle competition.

Successful relationships are collaborations between people in pursuit of mutually beneficial goals.

Relationship Management at Work

THE FOLLOWING IS A SAMPLE scenario related to relationship management involving RPG (recent pharmacy graduate):

RPG had gone to school later than most students. She was 37 when she graduated. Going to work in a large healthcare system, RPG found herself working for a supervisor who was 28 years old. RPG thought her supervisor was shallow and not really qualified for her position. More than that, RPG just didn't like her. She was not sure why, but the two of them just did not resonate with one another. RPG sensed that her supervisor felt the same way about her.

At a meeting of the pharmacy and therapeutics committee the supervisor was presenting her recommendations on the inclusion of a new drug in the formulary. During the presentation, RPG sensed that several conclusions that the supervisor presented were somewhat inaccurate. During the meeting, RPG Googled the drug and found support for conclusions that differed from what the supervisor said. RPG also noticed that some of her financial projections were based on exceedingly generous assumptions and ought to be challenged.

How would you recommend RPG handle the situation?

Assignment: What Do the Practitioners/ Others Say?

BE PREPARED TO DISCUSS RELATIONSHIP management based on any *one* of the following:

- A discussion with your colleagues, or others, on the concept of relationship management
- An article on relationships, either from the research literature or any other source
- A movie/television program/YouTube video about relationships
- A book on relationships (literary, historical, psychological, or any other source)

EXERCISES

⊪ Am I Active or Passive in Relationships?

Do you try to get along no matter what, or do you take charge of the relationship?

⫷ Your Relationship Foundations

How did your parents model relationships for you?

_____

How did your family respond to you when you communicated an emotional need?

_____

Were you encouraged to express your needs while growing up?

_____

If so, how? _____

If not, why not? _____

As a child, how did you get others to respond to your needs?

_____

As an adult, how do you get others to respond to your needs?

_____

Do your emotions get in the way of expressing your needs?

_____

How do you handle it when someone does not honor your request to have a need met? _____

Source: Adapted from Spradling, S. E. (2003). _Don't let your emotions run your life._ Oakland, CA: New Harbinger: 144–146.

⫷ Personal Learning Plan: Relationship Management

These steps can be compiled on a single page containing the following:

What prompted me to develop this plan?

What is the general area for improvement?

What is the specific issue for improvement?

Why is this important to me?

How do I generally act in these areas?

What are my goals?

What prompted this effort?

What strategies are required?

Who/what is necessary to meet my goals with this strategy?

How will I measure the success/failure of this effort?

How long will I focus on this effort?

How will I reflect and capture a lesson from this effort that can be generalized to other circumstances?

Based on your responses to the exercises, write a one-paragraph description of yourself as it relates to relationship management.

⁘ WHAT'S IMPORTANT TO YOU IN THE CHAPTER?

With several of your classmates, discuss the idea/ideas that are most likely to effect change in your values, attitudes, or behaviors. Be succinct—no more than two sentences.

⁘ REFERENCES

McKay, M., Wood, J. C., & Brantley, J. (2007). *The dialectical behavior therapy skills workbook*. Oakland, CA: New Harbinger.

Spradling, S. E. (2003). *Don't let your emotions run your life*. Oakland, CA: New Harbinger.

Tamm, J. W., & Luyet, R. J. (2004). *Radical collaboration*. New York, NY: Collins Business.

⁘ SUGGESTED READINGS

Didato, S. V. (2003). *The big book of personality tests*. New York, NY: Black Dog and Leventhal.

Fishbane, M. D. (2007). Wired to connect: Neuroscience, relationships, and therapy. *Family Process*, 46(3), 395–412.

Friday, P. J. (1999). *Friday's laws: How to become normal when you're not and how to stay normal when you are.* Pittsburgh, PA: Bradley Oak.

Goleman, D., & Boyatzis, R. (2008, September). Social intelligence and the biology of leadership. *Harvard Business Review,* 74–81.

Lipman-Blumen, J. (2005). *The allure of toxic leaders.* New York, NY: Oxford University Press.

Richo, D. (2008). *When the past is present.* Boston, MA: Shambhala.

Summary: Commandments for Emotional Intelligence

At the end of each chapter you were asked to list what was important to you in that chapter. Collect the statements for each chapter and review. Can any statements be combined, eliminated, or synthesized into simpler and more personally useful statements? The task is to arrive at the fewest statements that capture the essence of what is important and memorable. In other words, what are you likely to remember in 6 months, a year? Consult with your classmates on this exercise.

◀ WHAT'S IMPORTANT TO YOU IN THE CHAPTER?

Self-Directed Learning:

Emotional Intelligence:

Emotions:

Self-Awareness:

Self-Management:

Social Awareness:

Relationship Management:

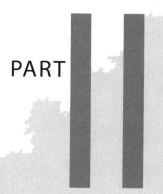

PART II

Professionalism

Professionalism is doing the best job for a patient you don't like, at a time that is inconvenient, on a day you don't want, while the patient is rude to you and you don't think you are going to get paid—because he or she needs you, and because taking the "high road" is the right thing to do.

The aspects of professionalism discussed in the following chapters provide specific markers of what it means to be a professional—accountability, altruism, duty, honor and integrity, excellence, respect for others, and the dark side of professionalism.

Ultimately, professionalism is about your character.

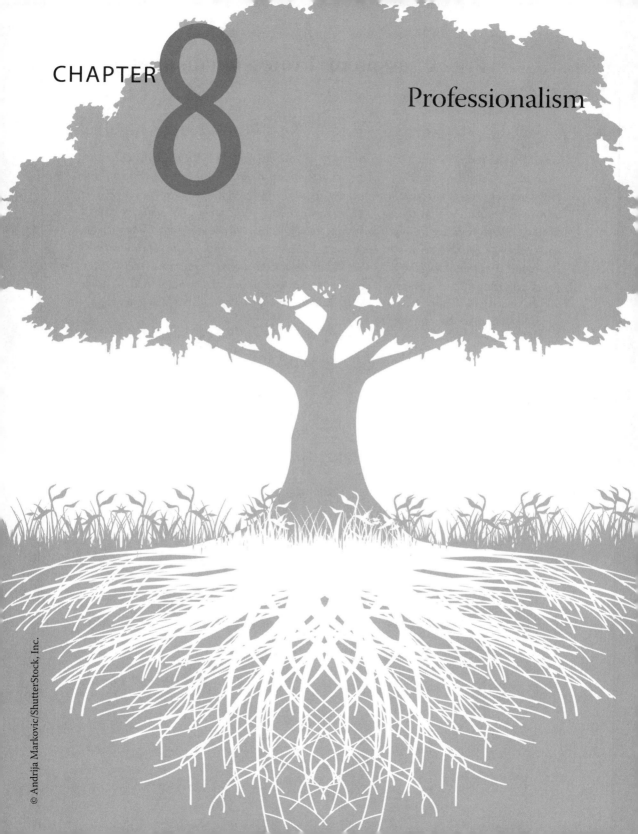

CHAPTER **8**

Professionalism

Pre-Assessment: Professionalism

Mind Mapping

Consider the term below. Without thinking or editing, write down the ideas, concepts, examples, contradictions, and theories that come to mind. Do not array them in any systematic or orderly manner. Scatter them about the page. Now, draw lines between your additions, indicating that there is a relationship between the terms. If something causes something else, indicate this with an arrow. Relationships may be reciprocal—both cause each other—requiring arrows at both ends. Indicate the strength of the relationship by darkening and thickening the lines—stronger relationships have darker and thicker lines. Most important: There is no right answer. Do not compare with your classmates. *What you have is a mind map, your mental representation of the topic. Review to determine if anything has changed following this section.*

Professionalism

⫸ DESIRED EDUCATIONAL OUTCOMES

- Describe the key elements of being a professional.
- Discuss the difficulty in developing professionalism.
- Discuss the impact of professionalism on careers and life.

⫸ DESIRED PERSONAL OUTCOME

- Achieve an enhanced personal level of professionalism.

What Is a Profession?

ACCORDING TO CRUESS, JOHNSTON, AND Cruess (2004), a profession is the following:

> An occupation whose core element is work based on the mastery of a complex body of knowledge and skills. It is a vocation in which knowledge of some department of sciences or learning or the practice of an art founded upon it is used in the service of others. Its members are governed by codes of ethics and profess a commitment to competence, integrity and morality, altruism, and the promotion of the public good within their domain. These commitments form the basis of a social contract between a profession and society, which in return grants the profession a monopoly over the use of its knowledge base, the right to considerable autonomy in practice and the privilege of self regulation. Professions and their members are accountable to those served and to society. (p. 75)

In summary, professionalism includes

- Mastery of a body of knowledge
- High levels of autonomy
- A code of behavior
- A social contract to do good for the individual and society

Who Is a Professional?

ANYONE WHO ADHERES TO THE standards of a profession and practices within that profession is a professional. "A real professional is a technician who cares" (Maister, 1997, p. 16). Professionals are people who do the best job they can on a day they don't want to, at a time they don't want to, with a patient they don't like even though they might not get paid—because the patient needs help.

What Is Professionalism?

DESPITE ALL THE WRITING ON the topic, the definition of professionalism is elusive. Professionalism is a complex pattern of values, attitudes, and behaviors. Although it can be broken down into its component elements, professionalism is a somewhat fuzzy concept. Professionalism is much like leadership, entrepreneurship, or being a true friend, an effective parent, an inspiring teacher, a great litigator, a quota-busting salesperson, an inspiring speaker, a great beauty, a learned scholar, or a world-changing innovator. The elements of all these are known, but only in their idiosyncratic expression can their true essence be captured and expressed. In other words, for each of these one can meet all the tests and possess all the skills, but something can still be missing. Professionalism is of the soul, an expression of character. Professionalism transcends the outward markers. It is not acting professional—it is being professional. Although your patients may see you as professional, your colleagues laud your professionalism, and your superiors count on your professionalism, only you, in the wee small hours of the night before you drift to sleep, know if you are a professional.

Professionalism is composed of our attitudes and behaviors. Our core values determine our attitudes. Attitudes predict our behaviors towards those elements on which our beliefs and attitudes are focused. If we see value in the dignity of an aging patient, our attitude will be positive towards this population and our behaviors will reflect this. If our values reflect the fact that all those people standing in front of our pharmacy are people with significant health issues, rather than an interruption to our day, or another insurance claim to be processed, then our attitudes towards those people will be positive and our compassion, empathy, and interactions will reflect this. Ultimately, professionalism is about how we behave.

What Concepts Are Closely Related to Professionalism?

Several other frameworks and constructs are related to professionalism, including professional ethics, professional commitment, professional responsibility, professional attitude, professional behavior, professional competence, professional values, professional identity/image, moral reasoning, work ethic, empathy, caring, advocacy, and covenantal relationships (Hammer, Berger, Beardsley, & Easton, 2003). These concepts are noted to indicate the lack of definitional clarity when discussing professionalism.

What Specific Behaviors Constitute Professionalism?

Specific behaviors related to professionalism include, but are not limited to, punctuality, appearance, courtesy, concern for others, grace under pressure, honesty, discretion, judgment, self-confidence, and commitment to excel.

What Values Are at the Core of Professionalism?

The core values that define professionalism include:

- A commitment to the highest standards of excellence in practice
- A commitment to the interests of patients
- A commitment to the needs of the community

These core values are elaborated as (adapted from American Board of Internal Medicine, 2001):

- *Altruism:* The willingness to serve the best interest of the patient rather than your self-interest.
- *Accountability:* This includes being accountable to individual patients in fulfilling the covenants of the patient/provider relationship, to society's health needs, and to the profession for honoring their codes of conduct.
- *Excellence:* A conscientious commitment to improvement.
- *Duty:* A commitment to serve the patient even when it's inconvenient.

- *Honor and integrity:* A commitment to the highest standards of behavior.

- *Respect for others:* A belief in the value of all human beings, including patients, families, and other healthcare providers.

How Is Professionalism Presented in School?

ALL STUDENTS BRING VALUES AND attitudes with them on entering school. Schools of pharmacy then undertake to socialize the student into the profession. This is an attempt to instill the knowledge, values, attitudes, and behaviors of the profession. The factors that influence this process are the culture of the school, specific activities delivered by the school, peers, and role models. While these activities are occurring students still spend approximately 75 percent of their time off campus. Activities and events in student personal lives also contribute to the socialization process.

Specific activities and initiatives aimed at fostering professionalism include the following:

- Introductory practice experiences
- Advanced practice experiences
- Experiential education
- Organizational initiatives (APhA/AACP/SNPhA, etc.)
- Selective recruitment and admission for professionalism
- Extracurricular activities
- Membership in student professional organizations
- Awards
- Mentoring programs
- Workshops/seminars
- Curriculum
- Mission statements

- Student handbooks
- Dress codes
- Pledge of professionalism/oath of the pharmacist
- White coat ceremonies
- Service learning projects
- Student portfolios

Do These Activities Work?

The activities that pharmacy schools deliver certainly provide students with a framework and anchor for their behaviors. Schools expose students to the desired professional behaviors so that they might model them. Activities provided by schools of pharmacy are, at best, only partially successful in developing professionalism and have been characterized as "not reliably effective" (Brown & Ferrill, 2009, p. 1). In medical education it has been noted that "medical training can disillusion and render cynical even some quite decent students, but rarely can it convert a basically self-centered and egotistical person into a humanitarian" (Glick, 1981, p. 1038). When schools of medicine were asked to demonstrate that their efforts at instilling professionalism were successful, the information provided "was at best apologetic and at worst oblique" (Hafferty, 2000, p. 16).

What Are the Impediments to Developing Professionalism?

There are several impediments to the development of professionalism. First, peer pressure in that other students, practitioners, and instructors fail to reinforce accepted professional behaviors or confront unacceptable professional behaviors. Second, the academic institution itself may be inconsistent or deficient in professionalism. Third, practice environments may reflect greater commercial aspects than professional standards. Fourth, practitioners the students come in contact with may be burned out, cynical, or jaded in their perspectives.

Why Is It Hard to Be a Consummate Professional?

SOMETIMES YOU WILL HEAR A colleague described as the consummate professional, meaning someone who conducts him- or herself professionally in all circumstances. Some professional behaviors are rather simple to acquire and exhibit, such as punctuality, appearance, and courtesy. Some behaviors are a bit more difficult to acquire and exhibit but should develop over time and with experience, for example, empathy, discretion, and grace under pressure. If not already present, it requires considerable personal insight, reflection, and work to genuinely acquire and exhibit the core values of a professional of altruism, accountability, excellence, duty, honor and integrity, and respect for others. The acquisition of new values is difficult because values are relatively fixed, though not immutable. These values just don't change overnight. Exhibiting a true commitment to excellence is not the same as putting on a clean shirt or blouse.

Why Is Professionalism Like a Religion?

PROFESSIONALISM IS MUCH LIKE A religion. Religions have codes of conduct, ceremonies, and respected elders and high priests. Professions have codes of conduct, ceremonies, and respected elders and high priests. Professionalism is the religion of the group of people you will be working with and for. Novices to the profession receive a code of conduct, a list of thou shall and thou shall not do certain things—in short, an aspirational declaration of how to behave. The student is baptized into the profession at a white coat ceremony and recognized into the profession as a full-fledged member, or confirmed, at graduation. Exposure to the high priests and elders of the profession, faculty and practitioners, models the appropriate behavior. Formal classes in professionalism can be viewed as religious instruction. The goal is to convert a nonbeliever into a committed practitioner of the professional religion.

How Is Professionalism Really Acquired?

THERE IS NO EXPRESS ELEVATOR to a pinnacle of professionalism. There is no book, no ceremony, no mentor who will speed this ascent from the ground floor to the penthouse. What is required is a commitment to a process of gradual improvement. Think of how a foreign language is mastered. Day after day, vocabulary, idioms, grammar, and the rules of syntax are acquired. Professionalism is similar. Gradually, the attitudes, values, and behaviors that constitute professionalism are recognized, understood, assimilated, and then woven into the pattern of our practice.

Why Should I Do the Extra Work to Be More Professional?

IF BEHAVING AS A NOMINAL professional will guarantee me economic security, why should I do the extra work, or extend myself to become a consummate, full-fledged practicing professional? This is the reason: All of us want to feel good—but, we want to feel good only if we are entitled to feel good as a result of our efforts and performance. Consider a group project in school. If the project got an *A* but you made a minimal contribution, the joy in the grade is diminished. The psychologist Martin E. P. Seligman (2002) relates an experiment conducted with his students. Each student was instructed to engage in one pleasurable activity and one philanthropic activity and report back. The afterglow of something pleasurable (a good dinner, a sporting event) is fleeting. In contrast, the impact of doing something good elevated the mood of the student for the entire day. Pleasurable activities lead to a hedonic treadmill, the continuous pursuit of pleasure where the bar for pleasure is continuously raised. Think of the progression in your thinking when you first started to drive. It may have gone something like this:

- Life will be sweet if I can just get my driver's license.
- Life will be sweet if my parents let me have the car this weekend.
- Life will be sweet if I can afford my own car.
- And at graduation from pharmacy school, life will be sweet if the dealer will just take another $1,000 off the new BMW I want.

The same pattern will repeat itself with houses, relationships, clothes, music, sporting equipment, or whatever pleasure you covet. In general, coupled with this hedonic treadmill is a tendency to compare yourself, your acquisitions, your pleasures to others. Continuously acquiring things will make for a pleasurable life, but not a satisfying one. The bottom-line message is this: "If you have the wrong values and motives, your life will not feel good regardless of how good it looks" (Krieger, 2005, p. 438).

In contrast, a satisfying life consists of using your strengths to pursue something larger than yourself and in the service of others. It is only by becoming a practicing professional, a fully engaged and committed practitioner of the profession's commandments, that one can be ensured of authentic happiness. The choice then is yours . . . to feel like an imposter in the sense that you haven't fully engaged your talents and strengths in the pursuit of others, or to be authentically happy by doing the work of becoming a practicing professional. Further, "Authentic happiness consists of raising the bar for yourself, not rating yourself against others" (Seligman, 2002, p. 14). In other words, a satisfying life derives from inner contentment, not external assessments.

Intuitively most of us would like to believe that those individuals who exhibit higher levels of professionalism will be more effective practitioners. We would like to believe that the energy and time spent to enhance our professionalism will result in tangible rewards. For lawyers, the conclusion is that there is "a significant positive relationship between an internalized high professionalism and . . . perception of effectiveness" (Hamilton & Monson, 2011, p. 23). Such evidence is lacking in the pharmacy literature, but there is no reason why the same relationship shouldn't exist for pharmacists.

Professionalism at Work

THE FOLLOWING IS A SAMPLE scenario related to professionalism involving RPG (recent pharmacy graduate):

RPG didn't mind working holidays. Most holidays were not that busy, and the extra money was always appreciated. It felt like the student loans would never be paid off.

RPG couldn't remember the last time she looked forward to a date as much as the one scheduled right after she got off work. She had just enough time to get home and get ready before her date arrived. They had dinner reservations at one of the city's most exclusive and hard-to-get-into restaurants. She knew she had to be on time. He was someone she was extremely interested in; someone with all the traits she was looking for in a permanent relationship. RPG thought, "I need to get out of here right on time," and planned to start the closing routines about 30 minutes earlier than normal to make sure she left as scheduled.

Five minutes before closing, a patient walked in with eight new prescriptions. It was clear that this person had just been dismissed from the hospital following a heart attack. The patient was alone and elderly. RPG could see that the patient had arrived by taxi. The patient was new, so all of the personal information, along with all the prescriptions, would have to be entered into the computer. Also, there seemed to be problems with several of the dosing regimens. RPG would not be comfortable dispensing these medications without confirming their correctness with the doctor. Call-backs from doctors often were not immediate. From the patient's address, RPG could see that he lived in the apartment building right next to the store and that this would be the most convenient pharmacy for him. In her mind, RPG calculated how long this was going to take—at least 45 minutes to an hour, because she knew her technicians would leave on time and she would have to do all the work herself. RPG considered telling the patient to go to a competitor pharmacy about 2 miles away that was open 24 hours. Her choice was to inconvenience herself or inconvenience the patient. RPG thought of her grandmother, who didn't drive and lived alone.

How would you recommend RPG handle the situation?

Assignment: What Do the Practitioners/Others Say?

BE PREPARED TO DISCUSS PROFESSIONALISM based on any *one* of the following:

- A discussion with your colleagues, or others, on the concept of professionalism

- An article on professionalism, either from the research literature or any other source

- A movie/television program/YouTube video about professionalism
- A book on professionalism (literary, historical, psychological, or any other source).

EXERCISES

⊕ What Is Your Definition of a Professional?

Most Admired Professional

Describe the most professional pharmacist you know. Provide a global description of what it is about their professionalism that you admire. Along with this global description, list several specific traits that define their professionalism. (If you do not know any pharmacist well, consider any professional in your acquaintance.)

Trait One: _____

Trait Two: _____

Trait Three: _____

For the traits listed, rate yourself in the following manner:

Trait One: I (routinely, sometimes, rarely) show this trait.

Trait Two: I (routinely, sometimes, rarely) show this trait.

Trait Three: I (routinely, sometimes, rarely) show this trait.

Most Admired Person

Describe the most professional person (in any area) you know. Provide a global description of what it is about their professionalism that you admire. Along with this global description, list several specific traits that define their professionalism.

Trait One: _____

Trait Two: _____

Trait Three: _____

For the traits listed, rate yourself in the following manner:

Trait One: I (routinely, sometimes, rarely) show this trait.

Trait Two: I (routinely, sometimes, rarely) show this trait.

Trait Three: I (routinely, sometimes, rarely) show this trait.

Least Admired Professional

Describe the least professional pharmacist you know. Provide a global description of what it is about their professionalism that you do not admire. Along with this global description, list several specific traits that are not admirable. (If you do not know any pharmacist well, consider any professional in your acquaintance.)

Trait One: _____

Trait Two: _____

Trait Three: _____

For the traits listed, rate yourself in the following manner:

Trait One: I (routinely, sometimes, rarely) show this trait.

Trait Two: I (routinely, sometimes, rarely) show this trait.

Trait Three: I (routinely, sometimes, rarely) show this trait.

Least Admired Person

Describe the least professional person (in any area) you know. Provide a global description of what it is about their professionalism that you do not admire. Along with this global description, list several specific traits that are not admirable.

Trait One: _____

Trait Two: _____

Trait Three: _____

For the traits listed, rate yourself in the following manner:

Trait One: I (routinely, sometimes, rarely) show this trait.

Trait Two: I (routinely, sometimes, rarely) show this trait.

Trait Three: I (routinely, sometimes, rarely) show this trait.

For both the positive and negative traits that you have identified and rated yourself on, ask colleagues and friends to rate you on the same traits. Do the external comments confirm your estimation of yourself? Try to explain the discrepancy, if any.

⬙ How Important Is It to You?

Please answer the following questions:

1. How important is it to you to be happy in your work? (very, somewhat, not)

2. How important is it to you to feel good about your work at the end of the day? (very, somewhat, not)

3. Is it possible to raise your level of professionalism? (yes, no)

4. How important is it to you to improve your level of professionalism? (very, somewhat, not)

5. How much effort are you willing to put into improving your level of professionalism? (significant amount, reasonable amount, not much, none)

6. Is your level of professionalism relevant to your career success? (very, somewhat, not)

Take a moment to reflect on your answers. Would it benefit your career if any of your responses were different? If so, how?

⬙ Professionalism Survey

Please complete the following using these responses:
SD = strongly disagree; D = disagree; N = neutral; A = agree; SA = strongly agree

1. I do not expect anything in return when I help someone. _____

2. I attend class/clerkship/work daily. _____

3. If I realize that I will be late, I contact the appropriate individual at the earliest possible time to inform them. _____

4. If I do not follow through with my responsibilities, I readily accept the consequences. _____

5. I want to exceed the expectations of others. _____

6. It is important to produce quality work. _____

7. I complete my assignments independently and without supervision. _____

8. I follow through with my responsibilities. _____

9. I am committed to helping others. _____

10. I would take a job where I felt I was needed and could make a difference, even if it paid less than other positions. _____

Answers that are agree and strongly agree indicate higher levels of professionalism.

Source: Chisholm, M. A., Cobb, H., Duke, L., McDuffie, C., & Kennedy, W. K. (2006). Development of an instrument to measure professionalism. *American Journal of Pharmaceutical Education, 70*(4), 1–6.

Based on your responses to the exercises, write a one-paragraph description of yourself as it relates to your professionalism.

❧ WHAT'S IMPORTANT TO YOU IN THE CHAPTER?

With several of your classmates, discuss the idea/ideas most likely to effect a change in your values, attitudes, or behaviors. Be succinct—no more than two sentences.

❧ REFERENCES

American Board of Internal Medicine. (2001). *Project professionalism.* Philadelphia, PA: Author.

Brown, D., & Ferrill, M. J. (2009). The taxonomy of professionalism: Reframing the academic pursuit of professional development. *American Journal of Pharmaceutical Education, 73*(4), 1–10.

Chisholm, M. A., Cobb, H., Duke, L., McDuffie, C., & Kennedy, W. K. (2006). Development of an instrument to measure professionalism. *American Journal of Pharmaceutical Education, 70*(4), 1–6.

Cruess, S. R., Johnston, S., & Cruess, R. L. (2004). "Profession": A working definition for medical educators. *Teaching and Learning in Medicine, 16*(1), 74–76.

Glick, S. (1981). Humanistic medicine in a modern age. *New England Journal of Medicine, 304*(17), 1036–1038.

Hafferty, F. W. (2000). In search of a lost cord. In D. Wear & J. Bickel (Eds.), *Educating for professionalism* (pp. 11–34). Iowa City, IA: University of Iowa Press.

Hamilton, N., & Monson, V. (2011). The positive empirical relationship of professionalism to effectiveness in the practice of law. *Georgetown Journal of Legal Ethics, 24,* 137.

Hammer, D. P., Berger, B. A., Beardsley, R. S., & Easton, M. R. (2003). Student professionalism. *American Journal of Pharmaceutical Education, 67*(1/4), 544–572.

Krieger, L. S. (2005). The inseparability of professional and personal satisfaction: Perspectives on values, integrity and happiness. *Clinical Law Review, 11,* 425–445.

Maister, D. H. (1997). *True professionalism.* New York, NY: Touchstone.

Seligman, M. E. P. (2002). *Authentic happiness.* New York, NY: Simon and Schuster.

⚕ SUGGESTED READINGS

Challis, M. (2000). AMEE medical education guide no. 19: Personal learning plans. *Medical Teacher, 22,* 225–236.

Chalmers, R. K. (1997, March). Contemporary issues: Professionalism in pharmacy. *Tomorrow's Pharmacist,* 10–12.

Chan, S. (2010). Applications of andragogy in multi-dimensional teaching and learning. *Journal of Adult Education, 39*(2), 25–35.

Pink, D. H. (2009). *Drive: The surprising truth about what motivates us.* New York, NY: Riverhead.

Sylvia, L. M. (2004). Enhancing professionalism of pharmacy students: Results of a national survey. *American Journal of Pharmaceutical Education, 68*(4), 1–12.

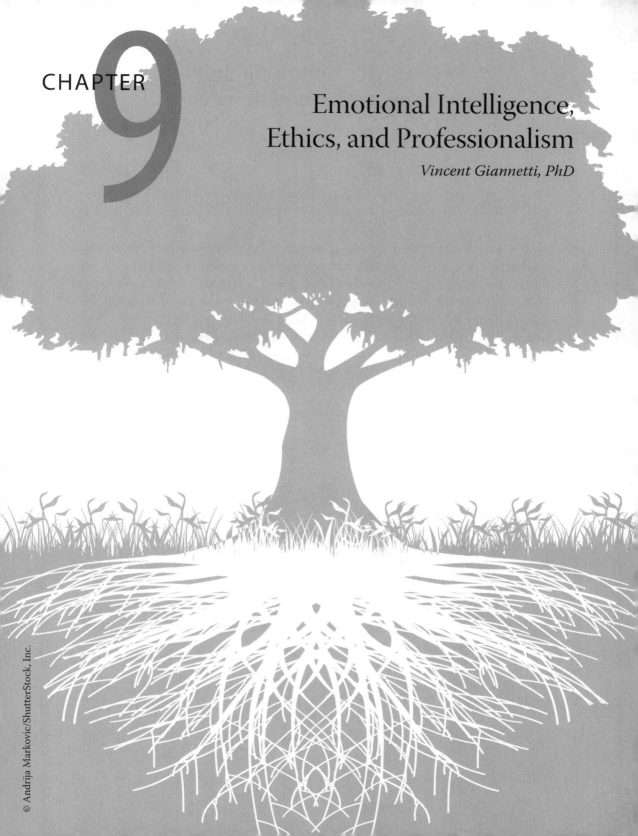

CHAPTER 9

Emotional Intelligence, Ethics, and Professionalism

Vincent Giannetti, PhD

Pre-Assessment: Emotional Intelligence, Ethics, and Professionalism

Mind Mapping

Consider the terms arrayed on the page. Without thinking or editing, write down the ideas, concepts, examples, contradictions, and theories that come to mind. Do not array them in any systematic or orderly manner. Scatter them about the page. Now, draw lines between your additions, indicating that there is a relationship between the terms. If something causes something else, indicate this with an arrow. Relationships may be reciprocal—both cause each other—requiring arrows at both ends. Indicate the strength of the relationship by darkening and thickening the lines—stronger relationships have darker and thicker lines. Most important: There is no right answer. Do not compare with your classmates. *What you have is a mind map, your mental representation of the topic. Review to determine if anything has changed following this section.*

Virtue
Ethics at work

⁕ DESIRED EDUCATIONAL OUTCOME

- Describe virtue ethics.

⁕ DESIRED PERSONAL OUTCOME

- Enhanced ethical behavior.

Learning Ethics or Being Ethical?

THE HALLMARK OF A PROFESSIONAL is his or her adherence to a professional code of ethics. All healthcare professionals have codes of ethics. In the case of pharmacy, the American Pharmaceutical Association code is aspirational in nature in that it declares the values of the profession without specific guidance regarding ethical dilemmas in pharmacy. The general field of biomedical ethics does provide a framework in the form of principles, theories, and methods for conducting ethical decision making (Beauchamp & Childress, 2009). Normative ethical theory in health care is prescriptive, focusing on what ought to be done based on applying specific principles to the facts of ethical dilemmas. These approaches are essentially intellectual and analytical, similar to doing problem solving in science and other disciplines. The problem with these approaches is that someone can learn ethics as an intellectual discipline without being able to consistently apply ethical behavior in professional practice. Put simply, knowing and doing are not always integrated.

What Is Virtue Theory?

AN ALTERNATIVE APPROACH IS CHARACTER development, sometimes referred to in ethics as virtue theory. Virtue theory does not focus on an analysis of specific acts, but rather on the development of character traits that predispose people to act intuitively in an ethical manner based on traits they have internalized. It is the proverbial acting ethically while no one is watching because ethical behavior becomes a habit or universal predisposition to act. This approach was best exemplified by Aristotle (384–322 BCE) in the classic *Nicomachean Ethics* and discussed by Annas (1995) and Pellegrino (2002). A detailed discussion of classical ethics is beyond the scope of this chapter. However, the important point of virtue ethics is the focus on the development of personal characteristics that allow for consistent, voluntary, and rational choices that aim for the ultimate good.

The approach of virtue ethics is based on personal development. Moral development progresses in age-related stages similar to cognitive and psychological development. This development begins with a simple reward/punishment orientation and then develops into instrumental morality, and finally, at its highest level, to a principled conscience orientation (Kohlberg, 1981). Acting on a set of consistent moral predispositions that are internalized and act as a guide to decisions in ethical dilemmas is the highest form of moral development.

Personal characteristics that make acting in a professional and ethical manner more likely need to be developed and acted on as matter of habit to facilitate ethical decision making. The standard principles in healthcare ethics are respect for autonomy, beneficence, nonmaleficence, justice, veracity, and fidelity. Although confidentiality is an important principle in ethics, Health Insurance Portability and Accountability Act (HIPAA) legislation has enshrined confidentiality in law, so confidentiality is now a legal obligation in addition to being an ethical principle.

In order to draw a distinction between an intellectual grasp of principles and a lived orientation toward acting ethically, the following example may be instructive. Consider for a moment a single mother with a sick child who has a prescription called in late in the day just before the pharmacy closes. She is not able to get to the pharmacy. Consider the difference between "going out of the way" to deliver the medication after you are done with work out of "duty" (an intellectual understanding of beneficence) or doing so out of compassion. Although the effect may be the same, what are the differences between how you interact with people when you are doing so out of duty versus genuine caring? Think of examples of when you do things for others or things have been done for you. What is the difference of doing or having someone do for you out of duty versus compassion or genuine caring?

Emotional Intelligence and Ethics

LET'S NOW REVIEW THE CONCEPTS in emotional intelligence and relate them to the standard principles in healthcare ethics. Emotional intelligence is a way of self-observation and active management of both personal psychological functioning and interpersonal relationships. It involves self-awareness, self-management, social awareness, and relationship management (Salovey and Mayer, 1990). To act ethically and professionally in any given situation, emotions and perceptions must first be identified. For example, respect for autonomy is a foundational principle of ethics. Negative feelings and perceptions must be recognized and bracketed, and the need for control must be abandoned. We can never control other people in health care. All we can do is offer options and provide risk–benefit information. Not offering full and reliable information to people is a violation of veracity and a form of control. Knowledge is power and allows self-determination. Withholding information places people under your control and unfairly deprives them of self-determination. Secondly, if we allow personal negative reactions to influence us, the necessary condition of nonjudgmental acceptance in helping relationships will never be established. In addition to self-awareness, self-management involves adapting our responses to patients based on an awareness of their needs, not fulfilling our needs for control or affirmation. Social awareness involves committing to a therapeutic (helping) relationship involving understanding the needs of others and recognizing the dynamics that can either facilitate or hinder relationships. Relationship management skills allow us to continually problem solve in relationships, form collaborative relationships with patients, and resolve potential and real conflicts. All of the dimensions of emotional intelligence are involved in respect for autonomy.

The interlocking principles of beneficence and nonmaleficence involve doing what is in the best interest of the patient as well as removing real and potential harms. Developing a genuine interest and compassion for patients allows these principles to operate naturally. Pharmacists serve people who have health problems. They often can act with frustration, anger, and despair. Simply learning the skill of empathy is not enough. Although it is important not to overidentify with patients, it is necessary to feel with them: If I were in this patient's shoes, what would I be feeling? When I was in a similar situation, how did I feel? If I or someone I was close to was in this situation, how would I respond? There is no doubt that practicing pharmacy emotionally engaged versus emotionally removed does place increased demands on the pharmacist. Caring comes at a price, but allows compassion to guide practice and increases the probability that ethical decision making will fit the unique needs and circumstances of patients.

Acting justly with patients often means confronting stereotypical perceptions that we hold. How do our negative emotions regarding the "addict" shape how we provide or don't provide pharmaceutical services? Can we maintain commitments to patients when they are difficult, or we don't agree with their decisions, or they look and act differently than us? It is unrealistic to believe that we will like or agree with everyone, but can we still respect their dignity and fairly give to them what they have a legitimate right to expect? Take your most attractive and likeable patient or personal friend and ask, "Can I act the same way with all patients regardless of their status or behavior?"

The essential core of emotional intelligence is the process of becoming self-aware, managing your emotions and perceptions, and becoming aware of others as distinct persons independent of your needs. Emotional intelligence involves learning to commit to relationships when they can be difficult and frustrating, manage conflict, form collaborations, and remain with relationships until ethical dilemmas are resolved. It is important to note here that although these characteristics are important for personal relationships, they are essential for professional relationships. In professional relationships the burden shifts to you to a greater extent because professionals function solely to serve the needs of the patient, not their own needs. This is usually not the case in personal relationships. The process of developing the skills and personal characteristics involved with emotional intelligence, along with an intellectual understanding of the theories, methods, and principles of biomedical ethics, will provide a strong foundation for professional and ethical practice.

Ethics at Work

THE FOLLOWING IS A SAMPLE scenario related to ethics involving RPG (recent pharmacy graduate):

RPG found herself working at a major health system that was extremely successful and well funded. By far, it was the dominant health system in the metropolitan area. The system has a policy of not loaning drugs to other hospitals and health systems if a drug was in short supply. On Saturday RPG received a phone call from a rural hospital approximately 50 miles away. The calling pharmacist said they had a child who was scheduled for surgery on Monday morning and required a drug that was hard to obtain due to manufacturer issues and asked if RPG would loan them enough for the procedure. RPG knew there had been some problems obtaining the drug, but because the health system she worked for was so dominant they always got most of their orders filled while other hospitals could only get one or two, if any. The calling pharmacist said transporting the child to a different hospital would create a significant hardship on the child's parent.

How would you recommend RPG handle the situation?

What Do the Practitioners/Others Say?

B E PREPARED TO DISCUSS ETHICS based on any *one* of the following:

- A discussion with your colleagues, or others, on the concept of ethics
- An article on ethics, either from the research literature or any other source
- A movie/television program/YouTube video about ethics
- A book on ethics (literary, historical, psychological, or any other source)

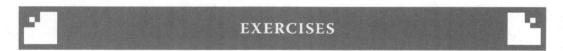

EXERCISES

Define the terms *autonomy*, *beneficence*, *nonmaleficence*, *justice*, and *veracity*. You can use any source, but put the definitions in your own words.

⑈ Ethical Transgressions

Identify and describe a situation where you have done or been tempted to do something unethical or illegal related to work in a pharmacy or any work experience. If this is not possible, relate a similar situation from your personal life.

⊪ Ethics, Professionalism, and the Emotional Intelligence Framework

It is highly unlikely that you have progressed this far in your career without being tempted to violate some ethical principle. The opportunity to deviate from accepted ethical norms will only increase as you age and you have greater responsibility and pressures to perform. Consider the situation you described above regarding doing something unethical or illegal, or being tempted to do something unethical or illegal as you read the following.

Self-aware: How did you feel in this situation? Did you change the way you acted? What emotions were driving this temptation? If you are doing something you believe to be unethical, do you have any behavior patterns that might give this away?

Self-management: What steps did you take to look at your emotions dispassionately and think rationally about the outcome? What steps did you take to control or manage this situation, both the actual event and the residual feelings following the event?

Social awareness: If another person was involved in this situation, what was going on with this person? How did he behave? What was the underlying dynamic for his behavior? How can you tell if he felt what he was doing was wrong?

Relationship management: How would you manage a relationship with someone you believed was doing something unethical? What circumstances would prompt you to report someone for doing something unethical?

⊪ Personal Learning Plan: Emotional Intelligence, Ethics, and Professionalism

These steps can be compiled on a single page containing the following:

What prompted me to develop this plan?

What is the general area for improvement?

What is the specific issue for improvement?

Why is this important to me?

How do I generally act in these areas?

What are my goals?

What prompted this effort?

What strategies are required?

Who/what is necessary to meet my goals with this strategy?

How will I measure the success/failure of this effort?

How long will I focus on this effort?

How will I reflect and capture a lesson from this effort that can be generalized to other circumstances?

Based on your responses to the exercises, write a one-paragraph description of yourself as it relates to ethics, professionalism, and emotional intelligence.

⚜ WHAT'S IMPORTANT TO YOU IN THE CHAPTER?

With several of your classmates, discuss the idea/ideas that are most likely to effect change in your values, attitudes, or behaviors. Be succinct—no more than two sentences.

⚜ REFERENCES

Annas, J. (1995). Virtues as a skill. *International Journal of Philosophical Studies, 3*(2), 228–294.

Beauchamp, T. L., & Childress, J. F. (2009). *Principles of biomedical ethics* (6th ed.). New York, NY: Oxford University Press.

Kohlberg, L. (1981). *Essays on moral development* (Vol. I). San Francisco, CA: Harper & Row.

Pellegrino, E. D. (2002). Professionalism, profession and the virtues of the good physician. *Mount Sinai Journal of Medicine, 69*, 6.

Salovey, P., & Mayer, J. D. (1990). Emotional intelligence. *Imagination, Cognition and Personality, 9*, 185–211.

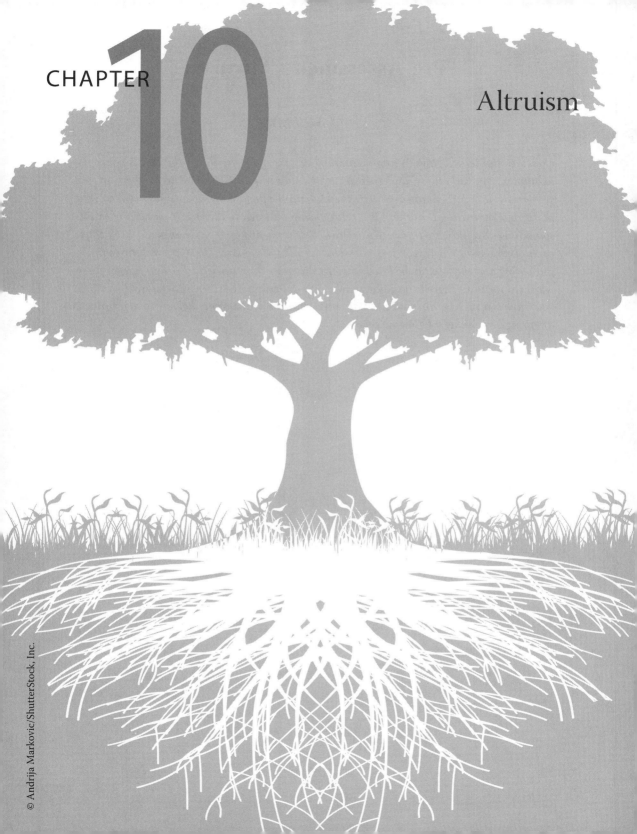

CHAPTER

10

Altruism

Pre-Assessment: Altruism

Mind Mapping

Consider the term below. Without thinking or editing, write down the ideas, concepts, examples, contradictions, and theories that come to mind. Do not array them in any systematic or orderly manner. Scatter them about the page. Now, draw lines between your additions, indicating that there is a relationship between the terms. If something causes something else, indicate this with an arrow. Relationships may be reciprocal—both cause each other—requiring arrows at both ends. Indicate the strength of the relationship by darkening and thickening the lines—stronger relationships have darker and thicker lines. Most important: There is no right answer. Do not compare with your classmates. *What you have is a mind map, your mental representation of the topic. Review to determine if anything has changed following this section.*

Altruism

⸬ DESIRED EDUCATIONAL OUTCOMES

- Define altruism, empathy, and compassion.
- List reasons for people being altruistic.
- Comment on whether you can be too altruistic.

⸬ DESIRED PERSONAL OUTCOME

- Increase the number of altruistic behaviors you perform.

"Altruism is the essence of professionalism. The best interests of patients, not self-interest, is the rule."

—American Board of Internal Medicine, 2001

What Characterizes Altruism?

ALTRUISM IS A SOMEWHAT VAGUE term. It is characterized by seeking to increase the welfare of another person rather than yourself. It is voluntary; the intention is to help another; and no external reward is expected. In many instances altruism contains an element of personal risk, for example, running into a burning building to save someone else's child. In the clinical arena this is seldom the case. A variation on the definition of altruism is "intentional and voluntary actions that aim to enhance the welfare of another person in the absence of any quid pro quo external rewards" (Steinberg, 2010, p. 249). Altruistic behavior is motivated by a desire to alleviate another's pain and suffering.

What Is Empathy?

EMPATHY IS THE ABILITY TO understand and appreciate how another person feels. Clinical empathy includes emotive, moral, cognitive, and behavioral dimensions. The emotive dimension is the ability to recognize the patient's perspective and understand their feelings; the moral dimension is the internal motivation to empathize; the cognitive dimension is the ability to understand the patient's circumstances; and the behavioral dimension is the ability to convey our understanding of his or her circumstances back to the patient (Stepien & Baernstein, 2006). In other words, I know how you feel and I can let you know it. Empathy is the understanding that I could be you.

What Are the Elements of Compassion?

COMPASSION IS MADE UP OF three interrelated elements. The first is the ability to notice the suffering of another. The second is the ability to feel another's pain, and the third is the response to another's pain and suffering (Kanov et al., 2004). Clearly, the concepts of empathy and compassion are very closely related. Although ethicists and philosophers devote considerable intellectual energy to drawing distinctions between empathy and compassion, for our purposes they will be considered to be synonymous. More important, we consider that empathy and compassion are at the core of and serve as the foundation for altruistic behavior.

What Motivates Altruistic Behavior?

TWO MECHANISMS CAN EXPLAIN ALTRUISTIC behavior. The first is termed egoistic—engaging in altruistic behavior will make me feel good and look good to others; in other words, I get something out of it. The second mechanism is pure altruism—I want to eliminate the suffering of other people without regard for my benefits.

Is Altruism Innate?

ARE HUMANS HARD-WIRED TO BE altruistic? Do we all come into the world with the capacity for altruism? There is strong evidence that altruism is an innate human capacity. It has been shown that newborns and infants will cry when other babies cry, which is construed as a primitive form of empathy. From an evolutionary perspective, altruism increases the chances for survival. Although an individual who is altruistic without reciprocation is disadvantaged, a group with high levels of altruistic behavior has greater chances of survival. Studies of twins suggest that a significant percentage of variability in altruistic behavior is genetic. Brain studies have shown altruistic behaviors can be linked to specific areas of the prefrontal cortex. In short, there is strong evidence that altruism is an innate human capacity.

Can Altruism Be Learned?

THE HUMAN BRAIN IS PLASTIC. Brain growth and learning are possible over a lifetime. Further, mirror neurons have been linked with empathy. Linking these two ideas suggests that growth in empathy and altruism is indeed possible. As with any behavioral pattern, there is always a choice. His Holiness the Dalai Lama contends that people can be either compassionate or not; in the end it is all personal choice. Quite simply, students can choose to be altruistic, just as they can choose not to cheat on a test.

Must Altruism Be Grand?

ALTRUISM DOES NOT REQUIRE GRAND, life-risking behavior such as falling on a hand grenade. Simple, thoughtful gestures suffice, as when a nurse sits down to share a popsicle and intimate stories with a cancer patient to acknowledge and ease the nausea and discomfort of a chemotherapy treatment. For the pharmacist, taking time to tell a first-time mother confronting her child's first ear infection that it will be OK, and that she is doing a fine job as a mother, is priceless. As Mother Teresa observed, "I never will understand all the good that a simple smile can accomplish."

Box 10.1   For Students, What Factors Affect Empathy and Altruism?

The following personal connections, experiences, and beliefs have been identified by students as promoting empathy:

- Past experiences
- Sharing of personal experiences and connecting with others
- Emotional intelligence
- General maturity
- Becoming a patient myself
- Having an illness in a family member or close friend
- Seeing patients die
- Having outlets and coping skills to deal with the aftermath
- Self-awareness and reflection
- Witnessing a patient's suffering
- Personal experiences with death and dying
- Upbringing and personal values
- Personal relationships
- Patient feedback
- Personal life issues and struggles
- Personal life changes and transitions

The following mentoring and clinical experiences have been reported to promote professional growth:

- Having determination to be empathic
- Increased understanding of our role in patients' lives
- Directly and significantly changing a patient's life
- Personal history of the same medical diagnosis as the patient
- Remembering why I chose this field
- Culture, race, and exposure to different perspectives
- Treating a patient with whom you have a lot in common
- Listening
- Exposure to people in need

Source: Adapted from Winseman, J., Malik, A., Morrision, J., & Balkoski, V. (2009). Students' views on factors affecting empathy in medical education. *Academic Psychiatry, 33*(6), 486.

Altruism as Marketing

PATIENTS WANT THEIR PHARMACIST, AND their other healthcare providers, to understand what they are going through and care for them—not in a clinical sense, but in a human sense. Viewed from a marketing perspective, rather than a professional one, empathy is one of five significant dimensions of service quality. The other service quality dimensions are reliability, responsiveness, assurance, and the tangibles (for example, décor, lighting). Higher service quality ratings translate into long-term relationships, higher patient retention, and increased revenues and profits. Although altruism asks the professional to consider the patient first, a byproduct of that professional behavior may be an indirect commercial benefit. In this scenario, no professional standards are violated. In the business world it is often said that "You can do good [financially] by doing good."

Why Is Altruism Good for You?

MOST INFANTS AND SMALL CHILDREN are the center of their world and their parents' world. With maturity comes an understanding that you are no longer the center of the universe and the selfish pursuit of personal happiness is futile. It is impossible to acquire enough attention and things to make yourself authentically happy. With maturity, the search for selfish fulfillment is replaced by an awareness of others' needs and your power to address these needs. Altruistic emotions and behaviors have been shown to positively impact mental health and physical health. "Altruism results in deeper and more positive social integration, distraction from personal problems and the anxiety of self-preoccupation, enhanced meaning and purpose as related to well-being, a more active lifestyle that counters cultural pressures toward isolated passivity, and the presence of positive emotions such as kindness that displace harmful negative emotions" (Post, 2005, p. 70). Similar to the saying in the previous section, "You can do good [emotionally] by doing good." The wisdom of Proverbs 11:25 (Revised Standard Version) prevails: "A generous man will prosper, he who refreshes others will himself be refreshed."

Caveats Regarding Altruism, Empathy, and Compassion

BEING COMPASSIONATE, EMPATHIC, AND ALTRUISTIC requires an emotional investment. This emotional investment is termed *emotional labor*. Emotional labor requires the practitioner to display certain emotions as an aspect of their job; for example, calmness in the face of emergencies to quiet the patient, or sorrow in response to a death. These emotional displays involve surface acting (displaying the emotion without actually feeling it) or deep acting (actually experiencing or feeling the emotion). The possibility of emotional dissonance exists in that emotions such as disgust, annoyance, and frustration must be suppressed and supplanted with caring and concern. Over time, excessive emotional involvement with the patient along with emotional dissonance may lead to cynicism and burnout. Self-awareness requires that you recognize when this is occurring and emotional intelligence requires that you modify feelings and behaviors to maintain appropriate levels of professionalism and performance. If you can no longer relate to patients, or find that they all make you angry, then something needs to change before patient care is compromised.

Altruism at Work

THE FOLLOWING IS A SAMPLE scenario related to altruism involving RPG (recent pharmacy graduate):

In just 2 years RPG had come to care for many of her patients, especially older women who lived alone. Because RPG lived 500 miles from her widowed, elderly mother she tried to treat these patients with special care and hoped that someone at home would do the same thing for her mother.

The weather report began to scream about a huge snowstorm moving into the city later that night. The prediction was for the city to be gridlocked for the next 1–2 days. RPG knew that one of her favorite elderly women patients was due in the next morning to pick up her customary bundle of prescriptions and insulin. Reviewing the patient profile, RPG determined that the patient was probably completely out of several of her medications. Although the patient could likely delay her AM meds until later in the day, if the predictions for the impending storm were accurate, then the patient might not get the meds for 2 to 3 days. RPG called the patient and confirmed her suspicions.

How would you recommend RPG handle the situation?

Assignment: What Do the Practitioners/ Others Say?

B E PREPARED TO DISCUSS ALTRUISM based on any *one* of the following:

- A discussion with your colleagues, or others, on how they feel and what they know about altruism
- An article on altruism, either from the research literature or any other source
- A movie/television program/YouTube video about altruism
- A book on altruism (literary, historical, psychological, or any other source)

 EXERCISES

⫶⫶ Attitudes Toward Altruism

Do you believe potential pharmacy students should be required to demonstrate altruistic attitudes, values, and behaviors for acceptance into a program?

⫶⫶ Altruistic Behaviors

During the past 12 months, how often have you done any of the following:

Donated blood _____

Given food or money to a homeless person _____

Returned money to a cashier after getting too much change _____

Allowed a stranger to go ahead of you in line _____

Done volunteer work for charity _____

Given money to a charity _____

Offered your seat in a public place to a stranger who was standing _____

Given directions to a stranger _____

Let someone you didn't know well borrow an item of some value _____

Review the number of altruistic acts on your part over the past year. What does this number suggest about your levels of altruism? Compare your numbers to several of your classmates'.

Source: Adapted from Smith, T. W. (2006). *Altruism and empathy in America: Trends and correlates*. Chicago, IL: National Opinion Research Center, University of Chicago: 42.

⫼ Revised Jefferson Scale of Physician Empathy (Adapted for Pharmacy Students)

Please answer these questions using the following scale:
1 = strongly disagree; 2 = somewhat disagree; 3 = disagree; 4 = neither agree nor disagree; 5 = agree; 6 = somewhat agree; 7 = strongly agree

1. An important component of the relationship with my patients is my understanding of the emotional status of the patients and their families. _____

2. I try to understand what is going on in my patients' minds by paying attention to their nonverbal cues and body language. _____

3. I believe that empathy is an important therapeutic factor in medical treatment. _____

4. Empathy is a therapeutic skill without which my success as a pharmacist would be limited. _____

5. My understanding of my patients' feelings gives them a sense of validation that is therapeutic in its own right. _____

6. My patients feel better when I understand their feelings. _____

7. I consider understanding my patients' body language as important as verbal communication in pharmacist–patient relationships. _____

8. I try to imagine myself in my patients' shoes when providing care to them. _____

9. I have a good sense of humor, which I think contributes to a better clinical outcome. _____

10. I try to think like my patients in order to render better care. _____

Source: Hojat, M., Gonnella, J. S., Nasca, T. J., Mangione, S., Vergare, M., & Magee, M. (2002). Physician empathy: Definition, components, measurement, and relationship to gender and specialty. *American Journal of Psychiatry, 159*(9), 1566.

⫴ Altruism and the Emotional Intelligence Framework

1. In your mind's eye, visualize the most important person (MIP) in your life. Who is he or she? What about them makes them your most important person? What specific traits, behaviors, and features make them most important?

2. In your mind's eye, visualize the most objectionable patient (MOP) you can imagine. Who is he or she? What about them makes them objectionable? What specific traits, behaviors, and features make them objectionable?

3. Emotional intelligence is the ability to understand your emotions as well as the emotions of another person, and then craft a behavior appropriate to the context. For the four emotional intelligence dimensions listed here, answer the associated questions.

   Self-aware: List and describe the feelings that your MIP and MOP arouse in you. Are any patients "hot buttons" for you?

   Self-management: Do you override your feelings in dealing with your MOP? Have you ever subtly or overtly displayed your displeasure with your MOP?

   Social awareness: List the aspects of your MIP and MOP that you focus on when you see them. Do you see any negative traits in your MIP and any positive traits in your MOP? Can you understand your MOP's world?

   Relationship management: Relationships with your MIP should be easy. In contrast, relationships with your MOP are likely difficult. Do you treat your MIP and MOP with the same level of altruism?

⫸ Personal Learning Plan: Altruism

These steps can be compiled on a single page containing the following:

What prompted me to develop this plan?

What is the general area for improvement?

What is the specific issue for improvement?

Why is this important to me?

How do I generally act in these areas?

What are my goals?

What prompted this effort?

What strategies are required?

Who/what is necessary to meet my goals with this strategy?

How will I measure the success/failure of this effort?

How long will I focus on this effort?

How will I reflect and capture a lesson from this effort that can be generalized to other circumstances?

Based on your responses to the exercises, write a one-paragraph description of yourself as it relates to altruism.

⫸ WHAT'S IMPORTANT TO YOU IN THE CHAPTER?

With several of your classmates, discuss the idea/ideas that are most likely to effect a change in your values, attitudes, or behaviors. Be succinct—no more than two sentences.

⊪ REFERENCES

American Board of Internal Medicine (2001), Project Professionalism, Philadelphia, PA.

Hojat, M., Gonnella, J. S., Nasca, T. J., Mangione, S., Vergare, M., & Magee, M. (2002). Physician empathy: Definition, components, measurement, and relationship to gender and specialty. *American Journal of Psychiatry, 159*(9), 1563–1569.

Kanov, J. M., Maitlis, S., Worline, M. C., Dutton, J. E., Frost, P. J., & Lilius, J. M. (2004). Compassion in organizational life. *American Behavioral Scientist, 47*(6), 808–827.

Post, S. G. (2005). Altruism, happiness and health: It's good to be good. *International Journal of Behavioral Medicine, 12*(2), 66–77.

Smith, T. W. (2006). *Altruism and empathy in America: Trends and correlates.* Chicago, IL: National Opinion Research Center, University of Chicago.

Steinberg, D. (2010). Altruism in medicine: Its definition, nature, and dilemmas. *Cambridge Quarterly of Healthcare Ethics, 19*, 249–257.

Stepien, K. A., & Baernstein, A. (2006). Educating for empathy. *Journal of General Internal Medicine, 21*, 524–530.

Winseman, J., Malik, A., Morrision, J., & Balkoski, V. (2009). Students' views on factors affecting empathy in medical education. *Academic Psychiatry, 33*(6), 484–491.

⊪ SUGGESTED READINGS

Gyatso, T. (2003). *The compassionate life.* Boston, MA: Wisdom.

Joachim, N. (2008). Teaching the art of empathic interviewing to third year medical students using a fairy tale—"The prince who turned into a rooster." *American Journal of Psychotherapy, 62*(4), 395–418.

Mann, S. (2005). A health-care model of emotional labour. *Journal of Health Organization and Management, 19*(4/5), 304–317.

Parasuraman, A., Zeithaml, V. A., & Berry, L. L. (1985). A conceptual model of service quality and its implications for future research. *Journal of Marketing, 49*, 41–50.

Parasuraman, A., Zeithaml, V. A., & Berry, L. L. (1988). SERVQUAL: A multiple scale for measuring consumer perceptions of service quality. *Journal of Retailing, 64*(1), 5–6.

Piliavin, J. A. (2009). Altruism and helping: The evolution of a field: The 2008 Cooley-Mead Presentation. *Social Psychology Quarterly, 72*(3), 209–225.

Schantz, M. L. (2007). Compassion: A concept analysis. *Nursing Forum, 42*(2),48–55.

Simmons, R. G. (1991). Altruism and sociology. *Sociological Quarterly, 32*(1), 1–22.

Spiro, H., McCrea Curnen, M. G., Peschel, E., & St. James, D. (Eds.). (1993). *Empathy in medicine*. New York, NY: Yale University Press.

Troy, T. (2006). Patients rank doctors on confidence, empathy, other intangibles. *Dermatology Times, 27*(11), 18–19.

Wicks, L., Noor, S., & Rajaratnam, V. (2011, July 21). Altruism and medicine. *BMJ Careers*, 1–2.

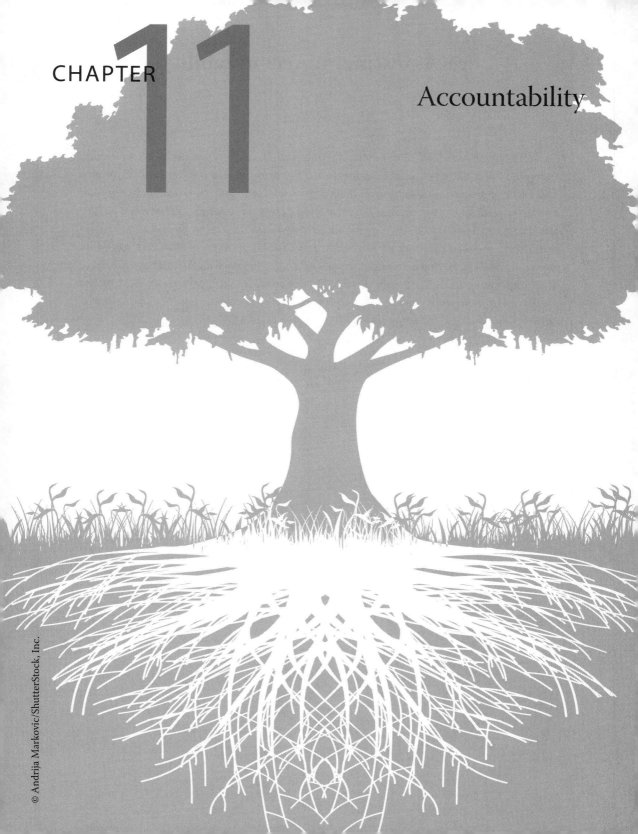

CHAPTER

11

Accountability

Pre-Assessment: Accountability

Mind Mapping

Consider the term below. Without thinking or editing, write down the ideas, concepts, examples, contradictions, and theories that come to mind. Do not array them in any systematic or orderly manner. Scatter them about the page. Now, draw lines between your additions, indicating that there is a relationship between the terms. If something causes something else, indicate this with an arrow. Relationships may be reciprocal—both cause each other—requiring arrows at both ends. Indicate the strength of the relationship by darkening and thickening the lines—stronger relationships have darker and thicker lines. Most important: There is no right answer. Do not compare with your classmates. *What you have is a mind map, your mental representation of the topic. Review to determine if anything has changed following this section.*

Accountability

⚜ DESIRED EDUCATIONAL OUTCOMES

- Define accountability.
- List the areas that professionals are accountable for.
- Discuss the psychological and emotional consequences of being accountable.

⚜ DESIRED PERSONAL OUTCOME

- Achieve an increased willingness to accept responsibility for professional deficiencies.

"Accountability is required at many levels—individual patients, society, and the profession. Physicians are accountable to their patients for fulfilling the implied contract governing the patient/physician relationship. They are also accountable to society for addressing the health needs of the public and to their profession for adhering to medicine's time-honored ethical precepts."

—American Board of Internal Medicine, 2001

Definitions of Accountability

THERE ARE A WIDE RANGE of definitions for accountability. "Accountability generally refers to the obligation of one party to be held responsible for its actions by another interested party" (Emanuel, 1996, p. 240). A definition of accountability from the business ethics literature is: "Accountability refers to the perception of defending or justifying one's conduct to an audience that has reward or sanction authority, and where rewards or sanctions are perceived to be contingent upon audience evaluation of such conduct" (Beu & Buckley, 2001, p. 59). Accountability consists of the people accountable to one another, the areas of accountability, and the process by which people are held accountable.

How Are People Held Accountable?

PEOPLE ARE HELD ACCOUNTABLE BY rules, codes of conduct, laws, and mechanisms of social control such as the expectations of important others. People also hold themselves individually accountable and suffer the pains of shame and guilt as a result.

Who Is Accountable?

HEALTH CARE IS AN INTERRELATED matrix of parties accountable to one another, including individual patients, physicians, pharmacists and other healthcare providers, hospitals, managed care, professional associations, employers, private payers, government, investors, lawyers and courts, pharmaceutical companies, and other providers of health-related products.

Box 11.1   What Areas Are Professionals Accountable For?

Professional and ethical accountability extends to multiple areas in a healthcare context. Those areas include:

- ❏ *Reliable delivery of care:* Is the right medication delivered on time, with appropriate directions and warnings?
- ❏ *Quality of decision making:* Are clinical decisions correct?
- ❏ *Confidentiality:* Is it maintained?
- ❏ *Fiduciary obligations:* Is the financial benefit of the patient paramount to ours?
- ❏ *Patient protection:* Are vulnerable patients protected?
- ❏ *Practitioner personal standards:* Are we competent, and do we remain so?
- ❏ *Equity:* Are services delivered equitably?
- ❏ *Cultural representation:* Are we sensitive to diverse populations?
- ❏ *Procedures for resolving disputes:* Do they provide procedural and distributive justice?

Source: Adapted from Emanuel, L. L. (1996). A professional response to demands for accountability: Practical recommendations regarding ethical aspects of patient care. *Annals of Internal Medicine, 124*, 242.

There may be other parties to this accountability matrix, but this list captures the predominant players. Accountability can be viewed through distinct lenses, including professional accountability (provider and recipient of professional services), economic accountability (consumers of health care as a product), and political accountability (citizens concerned with a public good).

What Is Attribution Theory?

ATTRIBUTION THEORY DEALS WITH HOW people justify their performance decisions. In other words, how do they explain the fact that they made a mistake? Attribution for the mistake can be related to either external sources or an internal deficiency. Internal attribution is a cognitive assessment that the individual was directly responsible for the event. Attribution for a mistake can be related to factors that were either controllable or not (e.g., although I can control my own performance, I can't control a patient's compliance to directions). Or, attribution for a mistake can be related to factors that are stable or unstable (e.g., being sick at work would be an unstable factor, whereas a personality tendency toward impulsiveness would be considered a stable factor).

Attribution also can be used to assign motive to other people. The same three dimensions can be used to explain patient noncompliance. Was their noncompliance due to internal or external factors, were the circumstances controllable or not, and are the factors permanent or transitory?

How Does Attribution Relate to Accountability?

ACCOUNTABILITY FOR POSITIVE OUTCOMES IS easy to assume. Accountability for negative outcomes is difficult. Accepting accountability for less than professional behavior, mistakes, errors, and deficiencies is difficult psychologically. No one relishes having to explain themselves in these circumstances. Psychologically it is much easier to explain a mistake if the attribution is due to external sources that were not controllable and not stable. Sub-par performance by healthcare professionals in New Orleans during hurricane Katrina would not be unexpected. Sub-par performance by healthcare professionals at a state-of-the-art facility, with adequate staff, during routine circumstances is problematic. Hurricane Katrina provides a psychological defense for sub-par performance. Sub-par performance at a state-of-the-art facility that is adequately staffed and occurs during routine procedures offers no such psychological shelter. Eventually, a professional has to confront the fact that they were, for the most part, responsible for the sub-par performance.

What Are the Psychological and Emotional Consequences of Accountability?

ACCOUNTABILITY IS AN ETHICAL AND professional obligation. Accepting responsibility for deficient performance generates emotional reactions, cognitive assessments, and behavioral reactions. Typical responses to accepting responsibility for deficient performance are:

- Shame conjures feelings of inadequacy, self-contempt, embarrassment, self-exposure, and indignity. Shame is a self-defeating emotion. Shame-prone people use rage, contempt, perfectionism, transfer of blame, denial, withdrawal, attacking the self, attacking others, and avoidance as defensive strategies to minimize their feelings. Shame focuses on the self. A shame-prone person would say, "I made the mistake because I am stupid." Shame is most likely felt when their transgression is made public, though shame may also be felt in private. Shame may be such an overwhelming emotion that the focus becomes the self rather than the person harmed. People who are shamed may try to hide or escape from the precipitating circumstance. Shame-prone individuals are more likely to blame external forces for their circumstances.

- Guilt is a transitory affective state arising from violating a standard. Guilt involves remorse, anxiety, and regret at having done something to hurt someone else. A guilt-prone person is most likely to say, "I did something stupid." Guilt does not have an element of personal self-evaluation; the focus is on the act. Guilt is typically a more private emotion. The feelings of remorse and regret are likely to motivate reparative responses. Guilt generates apologies, restitution, and seeking forgiveness. In contrast to the self-defeating defenses of shame, guilt is adaptive because apologies and restitution seek to repair and restore relationships. Apologies and restitution also alleviate feelings of guilt. True guilt comes from an empathic understanding of another person's distress and the understanding that our behavior caused that distress. Guilt-prone individuals are more likely to focus inward for the cause of their dilemmas. Guilt is a more developmentally mature emotion than shame. Guilt has the power to motivate reparative responses.

- Self-reproach is punishment for a mistake. Self-reproach involves an excessive sense of personal responsibility. Those who reproach themselves hold to an impossible standard with little concern for capability, circumstances, or individual psychology. The point of view is that there was an ideal response to a circumstance that I should have made. The reason I did not make this choice is, not that there was a momentary lapse, but that I am deficient.

From a psychological perspective, responsibility needs to be attributed accurately and realistically. "A clumsy focus on personal responsibility risks leading to self-defeating emotions like depression and overanxiety" (Nelson-Jones, 1987, p. 7). It is critical that the offending party does not needlessly erode their self-worth. Accepting responsibility for a deficient performance is only valuable if it results in improved future performance. Accepting responsibility is a professional obligation. Conversion of responsibility into self-blame is unwarranted and nonproductive. The best advice comes from the title of a book on managing medical failure: when confronted with inadequate performance, *Forgive and Remember* (Bosk, 1979).

How Does Personality Affect Shame?

CERTAIN ASPECTS OF INDIVIDUAL PERSONALITY may affect the emotional and psychological impact of accepting responsibility for deficient professional behaviors. The personality trait of perfectionism impacts feelings of shame. Perfectionism is either normal or neurotic.

A person with normal perfectionism is driven by positive reinforcement, typically a heightened sense of self-esteem and self-satisfaction. Those with normal perfectionism set realistic standards. Their perfectionistic behaviors are reinforced with praise, recognition, and feelings of accomplishment. When normal perfectionists fail they adapt their behaviors, change their standards, work harder, or simply accept the consequences.

In contrast, neurotic perfectionists set unrealistic standards that are bound to end in failure. Having failed, dysfunctional perfectionists have feelings of anxiety, depression, and inadequacy. They engage in avoidance behaviors. Neurotic perfectionists are not accepting of themselves. Failure is not an event, but an evaluation of their personal self-worth as a human being. Rather than addressing problems, neurotic perfectionists engage in excessive rumination on circumstances and tend to view the world in categorical black and white thinking. Those with greater tendencies towards neurotic perfectionism tend to feel higher levels of shame when found deficient.

What Is Self-Forgiveness?

TRUE SELF-FORGIVENESS CAN RESULT ONLY if the individual acknowledges the wrongdoing and their complicity in it. Self-forgiveness requires working though the attendant shame and guilt and arriving at a state of self-acceptance and self-respect. Self-forgiveness involves eliminating feelings of self-hatred and self-contempt. Those who can self-forgive recognize their intrinsic self-worth as being separate from an offending behavior. Self-forgiveness results in ultimately acting benevolently towards oneself rather than continuing to punish.

Accountability at Work

THE FOLLOWING IS A SAMPLE scenario related to accountability involving RPG (recent pharmacy graduate):

RPG loved her consulting work at the long-term care facility. Besides the heightened clinical responsibilities, she enjoyed the interaction with the patients, who were always happy to have someone new to talk to. Some of the patients had led such interesting lives, the stories they told. She also enjoyed that some of the male patients liked to flirt with her. She found their liveliness refreshing when compared to the status of some of her patients.

RPG had noticed that for the last several weeks one of her patients had been excessively agitated. RPG attributed this behavior to advancing dementia. RPG admitted to herself that she could barely get the charts reviewed in the time allotted. She was under pressure to pick up her newborn son from daycare by closing time. Being late picking her son up resulted in significant overcharges.

On one visit, RPG spent a few extra minutes reviewing the chart of the patient troubled with excessive agitation. RPG didn't know why she hadn't spotted the problem before. It was clear that the agitation was due to an inappropriate dosage regimen on one of the meds. The problem was easily corrected with a few notes in the chart.

RPG made the change in the chart and let it go. On her drive home she began to feel uneasy. What if the patient had been one of her parents? Had the nurses altered their attitude and treatment of this patient due to the increased difficulty in handling him? What of the doctor? Would his choices have differed if the patient had not been agitated? What of the patient's family? How were their choices impacted?

How would you recommend RPG handle the situation?

Assignment: What Do the Practitioners/ Others Say?

BE PREPARED TO DISCUSS ACCOUNTABILITY based on any *one* of the following:

- A discussion with your colleagues, or others, on how they feel and what they know about being accountable

- An article on accountability, either from the research literature or any other source

- A movie/television program/YouTube video about accountability

- A book on accountability (literary, historical, psychological, or any other source)

EXERCISES

⚛ Attitudes About Guilt

1. Briefly describe an event that made you feel guilty. If possible, focus on events related to your academic career or professional experiences.

⚛ Perfectionism Scale

Please answer these questions using the following scale:
1 = strongly disagree; 2 = disagree; 3 = neither agree nor disagree; 4 = agree; 5 = strongly agree

1. My parents set very high standards for me. _____
2. Organization is very important to me. _____
3. As a child, I was punished for doing things less than perfectly. _____
4. If I do not set the highest standards for myself, I am likely to end up a second-rate person. _____
5. My parents never tried to understand my mistakes. _____
6. It is important to me that I am thoroughly competent in everything I do. _____
7. I am a neat person. _____
8. I try to be an organized person. _____
9. If I fail at work/school, I am a failure as a person. _____
10. I should be upset if I make a mistake. _____

Higher scores suggest a tendency toward perfectionism.

Source: Stober, J. (1998). The Frost multidimensional perfectionism scale: More perfect with four (instead of six) dimensions. *Personality and Individual Differences*, *24*(4), 481–491.

ᐧᐧᐧᐧ Personal Responsibility

Take a moment to consider whether the following statements describe you:

I believe I am in control of my circumstances.

I believe that others are in control of my circumstances.

It is easy for me to accept blame and admit mistakes.

I believe it is up to me to make myself happy.

I tend to feel sorry for myself.

I believe I am in control of my feelings.

I tend to meet all my obligations on time.

In group projects I do my fair share.

I believe I am in control of my physical health.

I believe I am in control of my stress levels.

Based on your responses, write a one-paragraph description of yourself as it relates to accountability.

ᐧᐧᐧᐧ Accountability and the Emotional Intelligence Framework

Take a moment to consider a time when you were deficient in fulfilling an obligation. Were you late with a project? Did you fail to keep your end of a bargain? Did you neglect to alert somebody to something they should know? Have you ever disappointed someone with your choices?

Self-aware: List and describe the feelings associated with this deficiency. What did you think about? How did you behave?

Self-management: What did you do to control the feeling associated with this deficiency. Did you change your thinking regarding yourself? Did you alter your behaviors in any way?

Social awareness: How did other people react to you if they knew of this deficiency?

Relationship management: What did you do to repair any relationship impacted by this deficiency?

⊯ Personal Learning Plan: Accountability

These steps can be compiled on a single page containing the following:

What prompted me to develop this plan?

What is the general area for improvement?

What is the specific issue for improvement?

Why is this important to me?

How do I generally act in these areas?

What are my goals?

What prompted this effort?

What strategies are required?

Who/what is necessary to meet my goals with this strategy?

How will I measure the success/failure of this effort?

How long will I focus on this effort?

How will I reflect and capture a lesson from this effort that can be generalized to other circumstances.

⊮ WHAT'S IMPORTANT TO YOU IN THE CHAPTER?

With several of your classmates, discuss the idea/ideas that are most likely to effect a change in your values, attitudes, or behaviors. Be succinct—no more than two sentences.

⫸ REFERENCES

American Board of Internal Medicine. (2001). *Project Professionalism.* Philadelphia, PA: Author.

Beu, D., & Buckley, M. R. (2001). The hypothesized relationship between accountability and ethical behavior. *Journal of Business Ethics, 34,* 57–73.

Bosk, C. L. (1979). *Forgive and remember.* Chicago, IL: University of Chicago Press.

Emanuel, L. L. (1996). A professional response to demands for accountability: Practical recommendations regarding ethical aspects of patient care. *Annals of Internal Medicine, 124,* 240–249.

Nelson-Jones, R. (1987). *Personal responsibility counseling and therapy: An integrative approach.* Cambridge, MA: Hemisphere.

Stober, J. (1998). The Frost multidimensional perfectionism scale: More perfect with four (instead of six) dimensions. *Personality and Individual Differences, 24*(4), 481–491.

⫸ SUGGESTED READINGS

Borkowski, N. M., & Allen, W. R. (2003). Does attribution theory explain physician's nonacceptance of clinical practice guidelines? *Hospital Topics, 81*(2), 9–21.

Emanuel, E. J., & Emanuel, L. L. (1996). What is accountability in health care? *Annals of Internal Medicine, 124,* 229–239.

Fedewa, B. A., Burns, L. R., & Gomez, A. A. (2005). Positive and negative perfectionism and shame/guilt distinction: Adaptive and maladaptive characteristics. *Personality and Individual Difference, 38,* 1609–1619.

Hall, J. H., & Fincham, F. D. (2005). Self-forgiveness: The stepchild of forgiveness research. *Journal of Social and Clinical Responsibility, 24*(5), 621–637.

Parker, S., & Thomas, R. (2009). Psychological differences in shame vs. guilt: Implications for mental health counselors. *Journal of Mental Health Counseling, 31*(3), 213–224.

Rangganadhan, A., & Todorov, N. (2010). Personality and self-forgiveness: The roles of shame, guilt, empathy, and conciliatory behavior. *Journal of Social and Clinical Psychology, 29*(1), 1–22.

Shapiro, D. (2006). Self-reproach and personal responsibility. *Psychiatry, 69*(1), 21–25.

12

Duty, Honor, and Integrity

Pre-Assessment: Duty, Honor, and Integrity

Mind Mapping

Consider the terms arrayed on the page. For each term, without thinking or editing, write down the ideas, concepts, examples, contradictions, and theories that come to mind. Do not array them in any systematic or orderly manner. Scatter them about the page. Now, draw lines between your additions, indicating that there is a relationship between the terms. If something causes something else, indicate this with an arrow. Relationships may be reciprocal—both cause each other—requiring arrows at both ends. Indicate the strength of the relationship by darkening and thickening the lines; stronger relationships have darker and thicker lines. Most important: There is no right answer. Do not compare with your classmates. *What you have is a mind map, your mental representation of the topic. Review to determine if anything has changed following this section.*

Duty
Honor
Integrity

⬥ DESIRED EDUCATIONAL OUTCOMES

- Discuss the concept of moral reasoning.
- Discuss what a virtue is.

⬥ DESIRED PERSONAL OUTCOME

- Achieve a refined sense of moral obligation and moral intelligence.

"Duty is the free acceptance of a commitment to service. This commitment entails being available and responsive when 'on call', accepting inconvenience to the needs of one's patients, enduring unavoidable risks to oneself when a patient's welfare is at stake, advocating the best possible care regardless of the ability to pay, seeking active roles in professional organizations, and volunteering one's skills and expertise for the welfare of the community.

"Honor and integrity are the consistent regard for the highest standards of behavior and the refusal to violate one's personal and professional codes. Honor and integrity imply being fair, being truthful, keeping one's word, meeting commitments, and being straightforward. They also require recognition of the possibility of conflict of interest and avoidance of relationships that allow personal gain to supersede the best interest of the patient."

—American Board of Internal Medicine, Project Professionalism, 2001

"I am loath to close. We are not enemies, but friends. We must not be enemies. Though passion may have strained it must not break our bonds of affection. The mystic chords of memory, stretching from every battlefield and patriot grave to every living heart and hearthstone all over this broad land, will yet swell the chorus of the Union, when again touched, as surely they will be, by the better angels of our nature."

—Abraham Lincoln, First Inaugural Address, March 4, 1861

Why Is Lincoln Quoted for This Chapter?

Faced with secession and the splitting of the Union, Lincoln closed his first inaugural address with the previous quote. His appeal to prevent this dissolution rested on a belief in the "better angels of our nature," the best part of what it means to be human. He believed that ultimately this aspect of humanity would assert itself. Similarly, yoking someone with an obligation to duty, honor, and integrity is to believe in the better angels of our nature. A person who is dutiful, honorable, and resonates with integrity is virtuous, and that virtue is grounded in a personality that is anchored to their character. This chapter collapses the professional requirements of duty, honor, and integrity into a single notion of virtue, deals with virtue as an aspect of personality and character, and focuses on conscientiousness as the personality trait key to meeting these professional dictates. Duty, honor, and integrity bind the professional to an obligation for exemplary conduct, to an expression of their better angels.

What Is a Virtue?

Morality is the set of rules, doctrines, and lessons that delineates right and wrong behavior. Morality offers a solution to the everyday problems of life. Virtue involves conforming to these standards. Virtues express themselves in exemplary conduct. They are the characteristics valued by society. They have been extensively examined by moral philosophers, religious thinkers, and ethicists. This rigorous intellectual examination has confirmed their value. Some virtues are believed to be universal across all cultures. These virtues are believed to be grounded in biology and selected in an evolutionary process that is important to the survival of the species. The six universal virtues are presumed to be wisdom, courage, humanity, justice, temperance, and transcendence (Peterson & Seligman, 2004, p. 13).

Virtues and Character

Virtues are seated in character. Character is seen as the foundation of conduct. Individuals are born with aspects of character whereas other aspects develop over time. Character expresses the values and sensibilities of an individual. Good character results from an integration of personality traits organized around internalized moral values that are honed through practical application.

Virtues and Moral Reasoning

VIRTUES BEGIN WITH MORAL REASONING skills. These skills facilitate the distinction between right and wrong. Moral reasoning allows one to filter values, attitudes, emotions, and behaviors into good and evil. The predominant model of moral reasoning is Kohlberg's six-stage model. Those stages are (adapted from Kohlberg & Hersh, 1977):

Level 1. Preconventional Morality

Stage 1. Obedience and Punishment Orientation: In this stage children assume that rules are handed down by powerful authorities that must unquestioningly be obeyed. Morality is seen as external to themselves and punishment is associated with being wrong.

Stage 2. Individualism and Exchange: At this stage is the recognition that there is not just one right perspective handed down from on high, but that different people have different points of view. There is an element of fair exchange at this stage, of fair deals. Punishment is seen as a risk to be avoided.

Level 2. Conventional Morality

Stage 3. Good Interpersonal Relationships: As children enter their teens they move to an understanding that people should live up to expectations and behave in appropriate ways. Good behavior means having good motives. It also means having interpersonal feelings such as trust, love, and concern for others. Good attitudes are assumed to be expressed by the entire community. This stage works best in dealing with family and friends.

Stage 4. Maintaining the Social Order: At this stage the emphasis is on the community as a whole, respecting authority, obeying laws, and maintain social order.

Level 3. Post Conventional

Stage 5. Social Contract and Individual Rights: Here people begin to consider what makes a good society in a theoretical way.

People tend to believe that a good society involves a social contract in which all people have some basic rights that are best expressed through some democratic process. In this stage, morality and rights have some priority over laws.

Stage 6. Universal Principles: This stage is an attempt to define the principles by which we achieve justice.

It is argued that these stages are not simply the result of maturation; their development is not inevitable, nor are they the product of socialization. Rather, they develop from the individual thinking about moral problems. As the individual experiences more, and thinks more about circumstances, their moral reasoning is enhanced. A practitioner with a rich professional background and a sharpened moral perspective will understand what the virtuous choices are in any circumstance. Those choices then become the expression of their character. The goal of this process is the development of a moral intelligence. Interestingly, pharmacy students, when compared with a baseline of other healthcare professionals, have been found to ". . . be less morally developed than their counterparts . . ." (Latif & Berger, 1999, p. 20).

Is Moral Intelligence the Same as Emotional Intelligence?

EMOTIONAL INTELLIGENCE IS THE ABILITY to understand your own emotions and the emotions of another person, and then craft a behavior appropriate to the context. Self-control and conscientiousness require that we delay gratification, moderate dysfunctional impulses, and control our emotions in the pursuit of larger objectives. High levels of self-control, conscientiousness, and emotional intelligence are a prerequisite of virtue. The difference between emotional intelligence and moral intelligence is that emotional intelligence is neutral. Adolph Hitler and Jim Jones clearly exhibited high levels of emotional intelligence; however, their moral intelligence was obviously lacking. Moral intelligence takes the same skills and applies them to making ethical decisions and acting on them. Being fully aware of our emotions and their consequences is essential to cultivating emotional intelligence.

What Is Conscientiousness?

CONSCIENTIOUSNESS IS THE PSYCHOLOGICAL PROCESSES or mechanisms for expressing the virtues of duty, honor, and integrity. Empirical work confirms this link (Moon, 2001; Murphy & Lee, 1994). Furthermore, conscientiousness is one of the "big five" personality traits, which are neuroticism, extroversion, openness, agreeableness, and conscientiousness. Conscientiousness is the route to meeting the standard of duty, honor, and integrity. As a personality trait, conscientiousness is presumed to be relatively stable and general, but subject to variation due to circumstance. As such, conscientiousness can be elevated. The point is that more conscientious practitioners are more likely to meet and exceed the professional threshold for duty, honor, and integrity.

Conscientiousness is a global personality measure. It is related to or expressed as reliability, punctuality, assessing risk appropriately, planning, and being hardworking, persistent, self-regulating, achievement oriented, methodical, orderly, trustworthy, accountable, self-disciplined, well-organized, thorough, detail oriented, and careful. Intuition confirms the link between these measures of conscientiousness and positive outcome. In addition, empirical support exists for correlation between measures of conscientiousness and positive outcomes.

Self-Control as the Master Virtue

AN ASPECT OF CONSCIENTIOUSNESS INVOLVES self-control. In order to meet the professional obligation to duty, honor, and integrity, many impulses must be stifled. Lack of professionalism is often a deficiency in self-control. Some consider self-control the master virtue and the moral muscle (Baumeister & Exline, 1999). The process of self-control involves three activities: a clear understanding of the standards to be adhered to, monitoring of the self and keeping track of one's behavior in this regard, and a capacity to alter behavior to conform to the standard. Self-control is a relatively stable aspect of personality.

Self-Control as a Limited Resource

AS MENTIONED IN THE PREVIOUS section, self-control has been likened to a moral muscle. The executive aspect of the self, the ability to make decisions, interrupt behaviors, and initiate behaviors, rests on self-control strength. Self-control strength is limited; in other words, only so many impulses and urges can be constrained at one time. Undertaking a diet during study for the NAPLEX is probably not a good choice. This explains why small annoyances when one is stressed result in inappropriate overreactions. A flat tire on the day of a final evokes a completely different response than a flat tire the day after graduation. Muscles fatigue with exercise. Similarly, self-control fatigues with repeated use. Like a muscle, once rested, the ability to control oneself returns. Also like a muscle, repeated use of self-control increases self-control strength.

What Is the Deathbed Test?

ADHERENCE TO THE DEMANDS IMPOSED by duty, honor, and integrity lead to a sense of fulfillment, a measure of a good life. To determine whether an activity or choice leads to fulfillment it must pass the deathbed test. Although your career is just beginning, project yourself as being on your deathbed. Complete this sentence: I wish I had spent more time _____. It is unlikely any of you would respond with, working harder, making more money, reducing my golf handicap, or playing more video games. The likely themes are, with family, having a greater positive impact on the world, or being a better person. Duty, honor, and integrity are life descriptors that will meet the deathbed test of fulfillment, of having led a good life. Fulfillment requires effort, a conscious effort to adhere to the standards. It is not given to you. Being virtuous is a challenge for all of us; the personal costs can be high, but the psychic benefits of fulfillment, of a life well led, far outweigh these costs. Aristotle believed that virtue and human happiness are synonymous.

Duty, Honor, and Integrity at Work

THE FOLLOWING IS A SAMPLE scenario related to duty, honor, and integrity involving RPG (recent pharmacy graduate):

RPG was thrilled to graduate and be released from the pressures of school and NAPLEX. RPG planned to pursue residencies, most likely in psychology, with plans to go into academia. RPG knew he wasn't ready yet to take on the rigors of a residency, and returned to his hometown to work for a year in a small independent pharmacy. The pharmacist who owned the store had been RPG's inspiration to go to pharmacy school. He looked forward to a year of just going to work and spending a little money. Three months before RPG was scheduled to begin his residency, the pharmacist who owned the store had a stroke and was incapacitated. RPG knew the pharmacist needed the income from the store to support his care and the care of his family. RPG agreed to stay one extra year to help.

One year turned into 35 years, and now RPG is thinking of retiring. His wife has been having health issues and needs more of his attention. RPG is still in good health and still enjoys working, but she needs his help. The store and the small town where RPG has practiced for 35 years have been good to him. He has saved and invested enough to have a secure economic future. Over the past 35 years the town had settled into a gradual decline, with the population shrinking by half. Today the majority of the population in the town is elderly and retired. Over the same time span, the town had lost its doctors and was down to one elderly general practitioner who was likely to retire soon. The town has not been able to attract replacement physicians. In addition, the other two pharmacies in town have closed. RPG's store is the only one left.

RPG has been trying to sell the store for a year now. If the store closes, the next closest pharmacy is 30 miles away. This would be a real hardship for the elderly in town, particularly in winter. RPG has been talking to a new graduate for the last 3 months about buying the store. Being from the area, RPG feels this graduate is his last chance to sell the store.

How would you recommend RPG handle the situation?

Assignment: What Do the Practitioners/ Others Say?

B E PREPARED TO DISCUSS DUTY, honor, and integrity based on any *one* of the following:

- A discussion with your colleagues, or others, on how they feel and what they know about duty, honor, or integrity
- An article on duty, honor, or integrity, either from the research literature or any other source
- A movie/television program/YouTube video about duty, honor, or integrity
- A book on duty, honor, or integrity (literary, historical, psychological, or any other source)

EXERCISES

⦙⦙ Your Personal 10 Commandments

1. Take a moment and construct your personal 10 commandments. Although you may not have explicitly thought about it, you most likely have some rules that guide your personal and professional lives. For example, the first commandment: I would never cheat on a test even if I needed the points; second commandment: I would never cheat in a personal relationship; third commandment: I work out every day; forth commandment: I always prepare for class the next day before turning to recreation. Consult with your classmates on this exercise if necessary.

2. Speculate as to why pharmacy students would score lower on moral reasoning than other health professional students.

3. Review any of the YouTube videos of the 9/11 tragedy and the fire fighters who responded. How do you explain fire fighters being willing to walk into a burning building with a deep sense that they are about to die? What could explain this?

4. Would you accept a job knowing that if a better or preferred offer materialized you would take it?

5. Review the codes of ethics from various pharmacy-related organizations. Comment on similarities and the practicality of these codes.

⬥ Integrity and Self-Control

Please consider the following and rate yourself. How would others rate you?

1. Can you resist junk food?

2. Do you have a regular exercise regimen?

3. Do you live within your means financially?

4. Do you work as hard as you can in school?

5. Would you cheat to pass a test? The course?

6. Do you always keep your promises?

7. Do you do your share at work?

Based on your responses to the exercises, write a one-paragraph description of yourself as it relates to duty, honor, and integrity.

⬥ Duty, Honor, Integrity, and the Emotional Intelligence Framework

Was Lincoln correct, is there a "better angels of our nature"? Ask yourself, are people inherently good, or does evil dominate? Can people be counted on to do their duty? What about you?

Self-aware: Where did your personal 10 commandments come from? Who influenced them? How have they impacted your life? If you have trouble with this exercise, what does that say about you?

Self-management: What do you do when confronted with temptation in this area? How do you control your impulses? How do you handle transgressions of your commandments?

Social awareness: Pick a classmate—not one of your close associates. What do you think is one of their commandments? Can you tell from your classmate's behavior if they seem to be conducting their lives guided by some personal code of behavior? What clues indicate this?

Relationship management: Has violation of your personal code of conduct ever impacted a relationship? If so, how? What did you do to repair any relationship impacted by this violation?

⦀ Personal Learning Plan: Duty, Honor, Integrity

These steps can be compiled on a single page containing the following:

What prompted me to develop this plan?

What is the general area for improvement?

What is the specific issue for improvement?

Why is this important to me?

How do I generally act in these areas?

What are my goals?

What prompted this effort?

What strategies are required?

Who/what is necessary to meet my goals with this strategy?

How will I measure the success/failure of this effort?

How long will I focus on this effort?

How will I reflect and capture a lesson from this effort that can be generalized to other circumstances.

⦀ REFERENCES

American Board of Internal Medicine. (2001). *Project Professionalism.* Philadelphia, PA: Author.

Baumeister, R. F., & Exline, J. J. (1999). Virtue, personality, and social relations: Self-control as the moral muscle. *Journal of Personality, 67*(6), 1165–1194.

Kohlberg, L., & Hersh, R. H. (1977). Moral development: A review of the theory. *Theory and Development, 16*(2), 53–59.

Latif, D. A., & Berger, B. A. (1999). Cognitive moral development and clinical performance: Implications for pharmacy education. *American Journal of Pharmacy Education, 63*, 20–27.

Moon, H. (2001). Two faces of conscientiousness: Duty and achievement striving in escalation of commitment dilemmas. *Journal of Applied Psychology, 86*(3), 533–540.

Murphy, K. R., & Lee, S. L. (1994). Personality variables related to integrity test scores: The role of conscientiousness. *Journal of Business and Psychology, 8*(4), 413–424.

Peterson, C., & Seligman, M. E. P. (2004). *Character strengths and virtues.* Oxford: Oxford University Press.

⸬ SUGGESTED READINGS

Baumeister, R. F., & Exline, J. J. (2000). Self control, morality, and human strength. *Journal of Social and Clinical Psychology, 19*(1), 29–42.

Bradshaw, J. (2009). *Reclaiming virtue.* New York, NY: Bantam Dell.

Buerki, R. A., & Vottero, L. D. (2002). *Ethical responsibility in pharmacy practice* (2nd ed.). Madison, WI: American Institute of the History of Pharmacy.

Caspi, A., Roberts, B. W., & Shiner, R. L. (2005). Personality development: Stability and change. *Annual Review of Psychology, 56*, 453–484.

Coleman, R., & Wilkins, L. (2009). The moral development of public relations practitioners: A comparison with other professions and influences on higher quality ethical reasoning. *Journal of Public Relations Research, 21*(3), 318–340.

Dudley, N. M., Orvis, K. A., Lebiecki, J. E., & Cortina, J. M. (2006). A meta-analytic investigation of conscientiousness in the prediction of job performance: Examining the intercorrelations and the incremental validity of narrow traits. *Journal of Applied Psychology, 91*(1), 40–57.

Duncan-Hewitt, W. (2005). The development of a professional: Reinterpretation of the professionalism problem from the perspective of cognitive moral development. *American Journal of Pharmaceutical Education, 69* (1), 44–54.

Frey, W. J. (2010). Teaching virtue: Pedagogical implications of moral psychology. *Science and Engineering Ethics*, *16*, 611–628.

Hoerger, M., Quirk, S. W., & Weed, N. C. (2011). Development and validation of the delaying gratification inventory. *Psychological Assessment*, *23*(3), 725–738.

Janda, L. (1999). *Career tests*. Avon, MA: Adams Media.

Latif, D. A. (2000). The relationship between ethical dilemma discussion and moral development. *American Journal of Pharmaceutical Education*, *64*(2), 126–133.

Latif, D. A. (2009). The influence of pharmacy education on students' moral development at a school of pharmacy in the USA. *International Journal of Pharmacy Practice*, *17*, 359–363.

Moberg, D. J. (1997). Trustworthiness and conscientiousness as managerial virtues. *Business and Professional Ethics Journal*, *16*(1–3), 171–194.

Muravan, M., & Baumeister, R. F. (2000). Self-regulation and depletion of limited resources: Does self-control resemble a muscle? *Psychological Bulletin*, *12*(2), 247–259.

Roberts, B. W., Chernyshenko, O. S., Stark, S., & Goldberg, L. R. (2005). The structure of conscientiousness: An empirical investigation based on seven major personality questionnaires. *Personnel Psychology*, *58*, 103–139.

Tangney, J. P., Baumeister, R. F., & Boone, A. L. (2004). High self-control predicts good adjustment, less pathology, better grades, and interpersonal success. *Journal of Personality*, *72*(2), 271–322.

CHAPTER

13

Excellence

Pre-Assessment: Excellence

Mind Mapping

Consider the term below. Without thinking or editing, write down the ideas, concepts, examples, contradictions, and theories that come to mind. Do not array them in any systematic or orderly manner. Scatter them about the page. Now, draw lines between your additions, indicating that there is a relationship between the terms. If something causes something else, indicate this with an arrow. Relationships may be reciprocal—both cause each other—requiring arrows at both ends. Indicate the strength of the relationship by darkening and thickening the lines—stronger relationships have darker and thicker lines. Most important: There is no right answer. Do not compare with your classmates. *What you have is a mind map, your mental representation of the topic. Review to determine if anything has changed following this section.*

Excellence

⚜ DESIRED EDUCATIONAL OUTCOMES

- Describe the various aspects of excellence.
- Explain the two approaches to excellence.
- Discuss the concept of achievement motivation.
- Describe the meaning of deliberate practice.

⚜ DESIRED PERSONAL OUTCOME

- An improved and formalized approach to achieving personal excellence.

"Excellence entails a conscientious effort to exceed ordinary expectations and to make a commitment to life-long learning. Commitment to excellence is an acknowledged goal for all physicians."

—American Board of Internal Medicine, 2001

Excellence in What?

EXCELLENCE IS A RELATIVELY BROAD concept. The pursuit of excellence is facilitated by breaking the concept into three categories, technical, personal, and future.

Technical excellence involves the following (Kapur, 2009):

- *Evidence-based thinking and practice:* The critical appraisal of the quality, amount, and relevance of evidence required to make effective decisions coupled with judgment and common sense in the modification of that information in light of the patient's priorities.

- *Decision support systems:* Appropriate use of information sources spanning the gamut from simple search engines to expert systems with algorithmic formulas.

- *Effectiveness and efficiency:* Improvements in outcomes and cost-effective utilization of healthcare resources.

- *Learning and risk management:* Learning from experience to avoid repeating errors, learning new skills, and learning new factual information to support better clinical decisions and procedural competence. Risk detection and prevention involve steps to ensure that errors are minimized.

Personal excellence involves the following (Kapur, 2009):

- *Interpersonal skills:* Improved communication skills with patients and colleagues and expertise in the social and emotional aspects of practice
- *Collaboration and leadership:* Understanding the dynamics of working in a team as well as the leadership skills of directing and supporting
- *Resilience and stress management:* The ability to manage stress and persevere in spite of difficulties
- *Moral principles:* Adherence to the underpinnings of the moral enterprise of health care

Future excellence involves the following (Kapur, 2009):

- *Teaching and training:* Excellence in the development of future practitioners
- *Innovation:* The development of new knowledge, procedures, and treatments
- *Research and publication:* Enhanced research skills and competencies and their publication
- *Income generation:* The ability to generate grant support to advance the profession

These aspects provide a framework for the appraisal of excellence and avenues for improvement.

Excellence for What End?

THERE IS LITTLE ARGUMENT THAT excellence should be pursued, but to what end? In the pursuit of excellence the individual may be motivated by two different goals. The first goal is a performance goal—winning positive accolades and avoiding negative condemnations. In this context, achieved goals are measures of your ability. Conversely, not achieving these goals marks you as deficient. In this framework the individual may shy away from tasks that seem beyond their level of competence to defend their ego. This approach is about appearing smart. The second goal focuses on mastery of the task—increasing your competence. The second goal is a learning goal. With this approach, setbacks are seen as opportunities for learning rather than insurmountable obstacles.

Healthy and Unhealthy Striving for Excellence

THE PURSUIT OF EXCELLENCE INVOLVES striving for a type of superiority resulting from exceeding an external standard, besting a competitor, or surpassing a self-imposed standard. Pursuit of superiority where personal goals are aligned with societal goals is healthy. If the striving for superiority rests on feelings of inferiority, the goal may not be to complete a task but to dominate. Superiority is the objective, not the benefits derived from mastery. Hypercompetitiveness is a danger in this circumstance. Pursuit of excellence for this reason is deemed unhealthy.

Note that the pursuit of excellence, work ethic, and mastery are internal or intrinsic motivators, whereas status aspiration and the acquisition of money and wealth are obviously external.

Box 13.1   What Is Achievement Motivation?

Achievement motivation is the personal striving of individuals to attain goals. Achievement motivation is a concept that encompasses the following factors:

- ❑ *Work ethic:* Originating from the concept of the Protestant work ethic, this describes a motivation to achieve based on the reinforcement the work itself provides. It is a desire to work hard.
- ❑ *Pursuit of excellence:* Motivation that finds reward in performing to the best of one's ability.
- ❑ *Status aspiration:* Motivation based on climbing the social ladder, to dominate, to lead.
- ❑ *Competitiveness:* Motivation based on enjoyment of the competition with a goal of winning.
- ❑ *Acquisition of money and wealth:* Motivation based on material reward.
- ❑ *Mastery:* Motivation based on competition with oneself.

Source: Adapted from Cassidy, T., & Lynn, R. (1989). A multifactorial approach to achievement motivation: The development of a comprehensive measure. *Journal of Occupational Psychology, 62,* 302.

What Is Flow?

Flow is the sensation that people feel when they act with total involvement. The flow experience is one of enjoyment where people are fully immersed and concentrating, where time seems to fly. In flow, people do what they do for the sheer enjoyment of doing it, even at great costs to themselves. With the flow experience, people are absorbed in the activity. In this state people are motivated by the task itself. External rewards play no role in this experience. Excellence demands a heavy price in terms of effort and time. There will be no formal demand that you upgrade your skills. Excellence is more easily sustained if its pursuit generates the flow experience. In other words, it is easier to get better at something if you are inherently fascinated by the task and find enjoyment in it. It is not practice, or work, if you would be doing it anyway. This is not to suggest that those involved in a flow experience are not aware of the implications and rewards associated with that experience. There is always some proportion of motivation that is extrinsic.

How to Get Better

THERE IS NO EASY WAY to achieve excellence. Given a requisite base level of intellectual, moral, and personal intelligence, innate talent is probably not a deciding factor. Genetics plays some role, particularly in activities with a physical component. What is important, first of all, is a belief that improvement is possible—a deep belief in your ability to improve is the foundation. Next is a deep commitment to this process. Some have characterized this commitment as "rage to master" (Winner, 1996, p. 271). It has to be something you really want, to the extent that you will sacrifice innumerable other things to get it.

Commitment alone won't do it, however; it has to be coupled with practice, a specific type of practice termed *deliberate practice*. The most effective practice requires a well-defined task, at an appropriate level of difficulty suited to the individual, informed feedback, and opportunities for repetition and correction. Deliberate practice is designed to improve performance. It requires high levels of mental concentration. For example, shooting baskets is not deliberate practice; however, working specifically on follow-through after a shot, under the tutelage of a coach who films the activity and corrects it on the spot, while gradually extending the range until 500 baskets are made and crowd noises are piped in is deliberate practice. Concentration is the critical element of deliberate practice. Deliberate practice may not necessarily be fun, though some individuals might find it, or aspects of it, enjoyable. Even with deliberate practice, most people probably can't become anything they want to be, but with deliberate practice they can be more than they currently are.

The Role of Willpower

LIFELONG LEARNING AND THE PURSUIT of excellence require discipline and the willingness to forgo immediate pleasures for long-term benefit that is often little rewarded or appreciated by others. Only you know if you have done the best you can in a situation. Only you know if you are working at less than your capacity. Although your performance appraisals may still be adequate or even glowing, only you know if it is your best work. Only you know if your skills are starting to erode.

Lifelong learning in the pursuit of excellence requires willpower. The potential to improve resides in your willpower. You can control your thoughts through willpower. You can use willpower to control your emotions and your mood, your affect. Waking up grouchy does not mandate going to bed that night still irritable. You are most likely to be as happy as you decide to be. You can use willpower to control your impulses, to resist the temptations that continuously offer enticing alternatives to the hard work of doing good and being good. Finally, willpower can be used to control your performance, specifically, focusing ". . . energy on the task at hand, finding the right combination of speed and accuracy, managing time, persevering when you feel like quitting" (Baumeister & Tierney, 2011, p. 37).

Empirical evidence confirms that you have a finite amount of willpower that depletes as you use it, and the same reservoir of willpower is used for all tasks. Consequently, the caveat is that when you dip into the willpower reservoir it is best to focus on only one task at a time. For most of us, it is not that we don't have goals, but that we have too many of them. Willpower is enhanced by a focus, not on the minutiae of the daily task but on the prize at the end; not on laying the bricks, but on the cathedral that will result. Willpower is not about continuous denial; having met markers on the path to excellence, self-rewards are in order. It is not masochism that is of interest, but continuous improvement.

Excellence at Work

THE FOLLOWING IS A SAMPLE scenario related to excellence involving RPG (recent pharmacy graduate):

RPG was taken by surprise by the phone call. She had been wrestling with the calculations for a TPN for a newborn. She was absorbed for a few moments in the intellectual quest of meeting the multiple requirements for the child. The doctor on the other line was clearly frustrated and angry. He said he needed to have a calculation confirmed that he was not sure of. His tone and the urgency of the request caused RPG to lose her composure. She said she would call him back in just a few minutes. Unfortunately, RPG was not all that familiar with this particular problem. By the time RPG called him back, 20 minutes had elapsed. The physician thanked her for her help but told her he had taken care of it already; the sarcasm in his voice was palpable. As he was hanging up, RPG heard him say to the nurse, "That's the last time I'll call the pharmacy for help."

How would you recommend RPG handle the situation?

Assignment: What Do the Practitioners/ Others Say?

BE PREPARED TO DISCUSS EXCELLENCE based on any *one* of the following:

- A discussion with your colleagues, or others, on how they feel and what they know about the pursuit of excellence

- An article on the pursuit of excellence, either from the research literature or any other source

- A movie/television program/YouTube video about excellence

- A book on excellence (literary, historical, psychological, or any other source)

 EXERCISES

⫸ Achievement Motivation

Factor 1: Work Ethic

Hard work is something I like to avoid.

Yes _____ No _____

Factor 2: Acquisitiveness

If there is an opportunity to earn money, I am usually there.

Yes _____ No _____

Factor 3: Dominance

I think I would enjoy having authority over other people.

Yes _____ No _____

Factor 4: Excellence

I hate to see bad workmanship.

Yes _____ No _____

Factor 5: Competitiveness

I try harder when I'm in competition with other people.

Yes _____ No _____

Factor 6: Status Aspiration

I would like an important job where people looked up to me.

Yes _____ No _____

Factor 7: Mastery

I would rather do something at which I feel confident and relaxed than something that is challenging and difficult.

Yes _____ No _____

Source: Cassidy, T., & Lynn, R. (1989). A multifactorial approach to achievement motivation: The development of a comprehensive measure. *Journal of Occupational Psychology, 62,* 301–312.

Based on your responses to the exercise, write a one-paragraph description of yourself as it relates to your need for achievement.

⫸ **Excellence and the Emotional Intelligence Framework**

What do you believe all Olympic champions, class valedictorians, and Nobel Prize winners have in common?

> *Self-aware:* Describe an activity or an experience where you lost track of time. What kinds of things can you lose yourself in? What aspects of school, if any, do you find pleasurable. Would you rather be a wealthy pharmacist or a pharmacist respected for your skills?

> *Self-management:* Describe the thought process you use to "psych" yourself up to deal with the pressures of finals.

> *Social awareness:* Describe someone you believe meets the standard for continuous pursuit of excellence. What specifically do they do? It can be in either a personal setting or a professional setting.

> *Relationship management:* What would excellence in relationship management look like?

⫸ **Personal Learning Plan: Excellence**

These steps can be compiled on a single page containing the following:

> What prompted me to develop this plan?
>
> What is the general area for improvement?
>
> What is the specific issue for improvement?
>
> Why is this important to me?
>
> How do I generally act in these areas?
>
> What are my goals?
>
> What prompted this effort?
>
> What strategies are required?
>
> Who/what is necessary to meet my goals with this strategy?
>
> How will I measure the success/failure of this effort?
>
> How long will I focus on this effort?
>
> How will I reflect and capture a lesson from this effort that can be generalized to other circumstances?

✦ WHAT'S IMPORTANT TO YOU IN THE CHAPTER?

With several of your classmates, discuss the idea/ideas that are most likely to effect a change in your values, attitudes, or behaviors. Be succinct—no more than two sentences.

✦ REFERENCES

American Board of Internal Medicine. (2001). *Project Professionalism.* Philadelphia, PA: Author.

Baumeister, R. F., & Tierney, J. (2011). *Wisdom.* New York, NY: Penguin Press.

Cassidy, T., & Lynn, R. (1989). A multifactorial approach to achievement motivation: The development of a comprehensive measure. *Journal of Occupational Psychology, 62,* 301–312.

Kapur, N. (2009). On the pursuit of clinical excellence. *Clinical Governance, 14*(1), 24–37.

Winner, E. (1996). The rage to master: The decisive role of talent in the visual arts. In K. A. Ericsson (Ed.), *Road to excellence* (pp. 271–301). Mahwah, NJ: Lawrence Erlbaum Associates.

✦ SUGGESTED READINGS

Colvin, G. (2010). *Talent is overrated.* New York, NY: Penguin.

Demerouti, E. (2006). Job characteristics, flow, and performance: The moderating role of conscientiousness. *Journal of Occupational Health Psychology, 11*(3), 266–280.

Dweck, C. S. (2000). *Self-theories.* New York, NY: Psychology Press.

Ericsson, K. A. (1996). The acquisition of expert performance: An introduction to some issues. In K. A. Ericsson (Ed.), *Road to excellence* (pp. 1–50). Mahwah, NJ: Lawrence Erlbaum Associates.

Gladwell, M. (2008). *Outliers.* New York, NY: Little, Brown.

Sternberg, R. J. (1996). Costs of expertise. In K. A. Ericsson (Ed.), *Road to excellence* (pp. 347–354). Mahwah, NJ: Lawrence Erlbaum Associates.

Stewart, A. E. (2010). Explorations in the meanings of excellence and its importance for counselors: The culture of excellence in the United States. *Journal of Counseling and Development, 88,* 189–195.

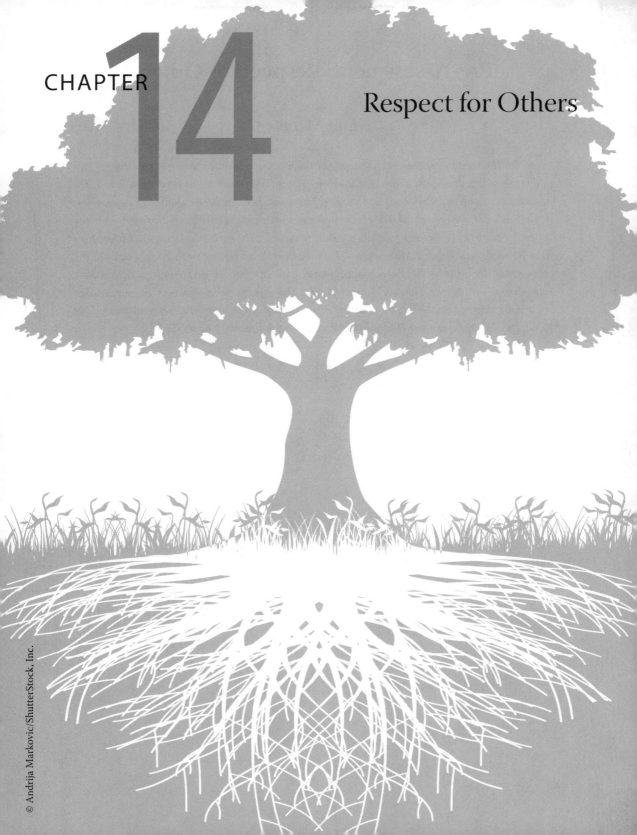

CHAPTER

14

Respect for Others

Pre-Assessment: Respect for Others

Mind Mapping

Consider the terms arrayed on the page. For each term, without thinking or editing, write down the ideas, concepts, examples, contradictions, and theories that come to mind. Do not array them in any systematic or orderly manner. Scatter them about the page. Now, draw lines between your additions, indicating that there is a relationship between the terms. If something causes something else, indicate this with an arrow. Relationships may be reciprocal—both cause each other—requiring arrows at both ends. Indicate the strength of the relationship by darkening and thickening the lines; stronger relationships have darker and thicker lines. Most important: There is no right answer. Do not compare with your classmates. *What you have is a mind map, your mental representation of the topic. Review to determine if anything has changed following this section.*

Respect
Civility
Cultural intelligence

❧ DESIRED EDUCATIONAL OUTCOMES

- Describe two aspects of respect.
- Describe the distinction between respect for patients and respect for others at work.
- Describe person-centeredness.
- Describe rudeness, incivility, and bullying.

❧ DESIRED PERSONAL OUTCOME

- Behave with greater personal respect for others.

Respect for others (patients and their families, other health care professionals, other staff) is the essence of humanism, and humanism is both central to professionalism, and fundamental to enhancing collegiality.

—Modified and adapted from American Board of Internal Medicine's
Project Professionalism, 2001

What Does Respect Mean?

THERE ARE DIFFERENT TYPES OF respect. One type of respect is based on an appraisal of an individual's worth; for example, we appraise someone as being a good person or a fine clinician. As a result, we believe the person is worthy of respect on this dimension. Appraisal respect is based on a comparison. As such, some people may be deemed not worthy of respect. A second type of respect is based on recognition of an individual's personhood. In other words, the fact that they are a person, no matter their status, conditions, or accomplishments, entitles them to respect and the behaviors that emanate from that respect. With this respect there is no comparison, no appraisal. This type of respect is due to all people, and due to them equally. This is a universal obligation of all people towards one another. It is this type of respect that professionalism demands, though it may be nuanced based on clinical circumstances. Although this respect is universal, it does not mean that all people are treated the same, because they vary in their needs and aspirations. In short, an unconditional valuing of patients as persons is the aspiration. This unconditional valuing of the patient as a person manifests itself in the idea of caring.

Respect for Patients Versus Respect for Others at Work

THE STANDARD FOR PROFESSIONALISM DEMANDS that all people encountered in the professional, clinical, and work context be respected. However, this demand varies based on the individual and their position and circumstances. The expression of respect due a dying patient is different than that due the chief executive officer of the health system, the chief of medicine, a fellow pharmacist, the administrative staff, technicians, and the driver delivering product to the pharmacy. Only with the patient does the pharmacist have the unique covenantal obligation that professionalism demands. With the others, the standard is not encumbered by these same standards. For the patient the demand is to care; for the others the demand is to be civil.

Person-Centeredness

ANOTHER WAY OF CONSIDERING RESPECT for others is through the idea of person-centeredness. Person-centeredness is a view that values people as individuals. Person-centeredness consists of the following (Coyle & Williams, 2001):

- *Personalization:* Treating the patient as a whole person
- *Empowerment:* Letting the patient have input into treatments and regimens
- *Respectfulness:* Issues related to seeing the patient as a unique individual
- *Information:* Keeping the patient informed
- *Approachability and availability:* Being there when needed
- *Life impact:* Considering the impact of the disease and treatment

Box 14.1   How Is Respect for Others Expressed in a Clinical Context?

Respect for others in a clinical context is expressed as:

- ❑ *Acceptance:* Accepting the patient as they are; where they are.
- ❑ *Advocating:* Being an advocate for the patient's rights.
- ❑ *Awareness:* Being aware of personal bias and the family and cultural dynamics at play.
- ❑ *Caring:* What can I do to help the patient through this?
- ❑ *Collegiality:* Discussing with other practitioners what the patient's feelings are and what they mean.
- ❑ *Communicating:* Clearly and appropriately communicating with the patient, both verbally and nonverbally.
- ❑ *Compassion:* A willingness to listen.
- ❑ *Competence:* Knowing how to ask the right questions and assess the situation.
- ❑ *Dignity:* Not taking the patient's independence away; attention to privacy.
- ❑ *Empathy:* Picture the patient's needs as primary, treating as you would want to be treated.
- ❑ *Justice:* Health care is justice due the other; respect is about equality.
- ❑ *Kindness:* Can I help? A sense of humor.
- ❑ *Presence:* Being there with the patient, being humble.
- ❑ *Reciprocity:* Viewing health care as a chance to give back all the good that has been given you.
- ❑ *Reflection:* Taking time to think how you could have done it better.
- ❑ *Relatedness:* Being able to engage with the patient.
- ❑ *Teaching:* Taking time to teach the patient what they need to know.
- ❑ *Time:* Not being rushed.
- ❑ *Touch:* A simple pat on the shoulder.

Source: Adapted from Maloney, R. J. (2009). *A phenomenological focus on Levinas' concept of alterity interpreted as respect for the other in a healthcare encounter* (Unpublished doctoral dissertation). Widener University, Widener, PA, p. 100.

Person-centeredness includes having a sympathetic presence. It is viewing the patient not as a case or a unit of production or revenue, but as a human being worthy of care and respect, regardless of their circumstances.

Rudeness, Incivility, and Bullying

R ESPECT FOR NONPATIENTS AT WORK is best framed by the negative aspects of rudeness, incivility, and bullying. Limiting these behaviors guarantees we will treat our coworkers and associates with respect.

- Rudeness is to disregard another. It is to diminish and demean. Rudeness invalidates the worth of another. It often emerges when people are stressed, unhappy, or rushed.

- Workplace incivility is ". . . low-intensity deviant behavior with ambiguous intent to harm the target, in violation of workplace norms for mutual respect. Uncivil behaviors are characteristically rude and discourteous, displaying lack of regard for others" (Andersson & Pearson, 1999, p. 475). Incivility includes not only verbal abuse, but also nonverbal behaviors such as glaring, ignoring, excluding, emotional aggression, berating via emails, taking credit for another's work, refusing to work collaboratively, withholding important information, gossiping, spreading rumors, and damaging a coworker's reputation.

- Bullying is a form of aggression. It is deliberate and repetitive. Bullying is ". . . repeated unwelcomed negative act or acts (physical, verbal, or psychological intimidation), that can involve criticism and humiliation intended to cause fear, distress, or harm to the target from one or more individuals in any source of power with the target of the bullying having difficulties defending himself or herself" (Bartlett & Bartlett, 2011, p. 71).

Rudeness, incivility, and bullying are measures of professional misconduct. Rudeness can be viewed as a precursor to incivility and bullying. On a scale from 1 to 10, incivility can be rated from 1 to 3, bullying from 4 to 9, and, though not discussed, battery and homicide rate as a 10.

Without question, rudeness, incivility, and bullying poison the work environment. At an organizational level they cause absenteeism, diminish performance, cause errors, promote turnover, and lower morale. For individuals, they increase stress and produce headaches, cardiovascular issues, anger, anxiety, and depression.

Advice on How to Treat People at Work

SOME OF THE BEST ADVICE on how to treat people was published more than 75 years ago. What follows borrows from that publication, *How to Win Friends and Influence People* by Dale Carnegie. There is nothing wrong with wanting people at work to like you; things go smoother that way. The secrets to this are:

- *Don't criticize, condemn, or complain.* Ben Franklin claimed the secret of his success to be, "I will speak ill of no man . . . and speak all the good I know of everybody."

- *Give honest and sincere appreciation.* The American philosopher John Dewey concluded that the deepest desire in human nature is "the desire to be important." Appreciation is sincere, it comes from the heart, it is unselfish. Make the other person feel important.

- *Smile.* It will make you and everyone else around you feel good.

- *Show respect for the other person's opinions; never argue.* You are most likely not always the smartest person in the room. Recognize the talents and views of other people.

- *If you are wrong, admit it.* No one gets it right every day. Knowing that you are wrong and admitting it is a mark of maturity.

- *Try to see the other's point of view.* It is just as valid as yours and just as strongly held as yours.

John Walker Wayland wrote in 1899 that a true man was one "who does not make the poor man conscious of his poverty, an obscure man of his obscurity, or any man of his inferiority or deformity: who is himself humbled if necessity compels him to humble another; who does not flatter wealth, cringe before power, or boast of his own possessions or achievements; who speaks with frankness but always with sincerity and sympathy; whose deed follows his word."

Cultural Intelligence

"CULTURE IS THE RELATIVELY STABLE set of inner values and beliefs generally held by groups of people in countries or regions and the noticeable impact those values and beliefs have on the people's outward behavior and environment" (Peterson, 2004, p. 17). "Cultural intelligence is the ability to engage in a set of behaviors that uses skills [e.g., language or interpersonal skills] and qualities [e.g., tolerance for ambiguity, flexibility] that are tuned appropriately to the culture-based values and attitudes of the people with whom one interacts" (Peterson, 2004, p. 89). A related term is *cultural competence*, the ability to accommodate variation in people and circumstances arising from cultural differences. Cultural competence in health care requires tailoring responses to meet diverse patients' needs. Like emotional intelligence, cultural intelligence is the ability to craft behaviors appropriate to the context, in this case the challenge of two people with different expectations and assumptions that are culturally derived affecting a positive health outcome.

Culture makes this difficult because only some of what we think of as culture is readily observable. Culture can be thought of metaphorically as an iceberg; like an iceberg, the largest part of culture is hidden below the surface. The cultural attributes readily observable include language, architecture, food, music, clothing, emotional display, gestures, and eye contact. Cultural attributes such as notions of time, the individual's role in society, beliefs about human nature and relationships, tolerance for change, passiveness, and others are hidden below the surface. The U.S. Census Bureau's 2012 *Statistical Abstract of the United States* reports that over 35 million people in the United States are foreign born. Cultural intelligence/competence is a required skill in meeting the test of respecting others, and an issue that no practitioner is likely to avoid.

Cultural intelligence requires knowledge about specific cultures, an awareness of yourself on this point, and the specific skills and behaviors to act effectively. Cultural intelligence can be thought of as a specialized type of emotional intelligence requiring facility in each of the four domains of emotional intelligence—self-awareness, self-management, social awareness, and relationship management. Similarly, the case could be made for a professional to be adept at generational intelligence, gender intelligence, and status intelligence: how age, gender, and status impact practice and health outcomes. The process of increasing cultural intelligence is the same as the process of increasing emotional intelligence. A person from another culture is not an exotic specimen beyond comprehension. He or she is a human being just like you, with feelings, emotions, and cognitive patterns. The task is to understand how their culture impacts those feelings, emotions, and cognitive patterns along with how your own culture impacts your feelings, emotions, and cognitive patterns and act accordingly—act professionally.

Respect for Others at Work

THE FOLLOWING IS A SAMPLE scenario related to respect for others involving RPG (recent pharmacy graduate):

> The old woman arrived in the pharmacy on a quiet Sunday afternoon shift, right before the Christmas holidays. With her was a young woman in her early twenties who was clearly developmentally challenged. She was there to have birth control pills filled for the young woman on Medicaid. She asked if she could talk to RPG. RPG said "Certainly." The woman relayed how she was old and knew she didn't have much time left. She said she didn't know what to do. She was the only one left to take care of the young woman. She was concerned what would happen after she was gone because she knew that the young woman "liked boys" and she knew the young woman could not be counted on to conform to any drug regimen by herself. She was also concerned that in a group home situation the young woman would be taken advantage of. If the worst happened, she knew the young woman couldn't take care of a baby.

How would you recommend RPG handle the situation?

> RPG thought the man was ancient. From his vantage point of a 24-year-old, an 86-year-old man was beyond comprehension. The old man asked to talk to RPG in private. At the time, the only private place in the pharmacy was a small room used for compounding. The old man relayed that he had cancer and that they were treating it with estrogen. He didn't like that they were feminizing him. The doctors suggested that the only alternative was surgical removal of the testes. He asked what to do. The old man looked like he was about to cry.

How would you recommend RPG handle the situation?

Assignment: What Do the Practitioners/ Others Say?

B E PREPARED TO DISCUSS RESPECT for others based on any *one* of the following:

- A discussion with your colleagues, or others, on how they feel and what they know about respect for others
- An article on respect for others, either from the research literature or any other source
- A movie/television program/YouTube video about respect for others
- A book on respect for others (literary, historical, psychological, or any other source)

EXERCISES

⫸ Civility at Work

Have you ever made fun of someone at work? Said something hurtful? Cursed at someone? Been rude to someone? Gossiped about someone? If you answered yes to any of these, how did this make you feel? How did you handle it? How would you feel if someone did the same thing to you?

Source: Adapted from Blau, G., & Andersson, L. (2005). Testing a measure of instigated workplace incivility. *Journal of Occupational and Organizational Psychology, 78*, 604.

⫸ Confidence in Cultural Competence

Please answer the questions using the following scale:
No confidence; Somewhat confident; Complete confidence

    Confidence that you can elicit patients' opinions, beliefs, and values about medications and treatment when counseling a patient

    _____

    Confidence that you can elicit patients' beliefs about their health and illness _____

Confidence that you can elicit patients' customs and healing traditions
_____

Confidence that you can assess the presence of language barriers
_____

Confidence that you can assess patients' literacy skills
_____

Confidence that you can acknowledge the diverse health beliefs of your patients _____

Confidence that you can elicit how patients' health decisions are made _____

Confidence that you can develop rapport with all patients regardless of their cultural background _____

Confidence that you can communicate to patients your understanding regarding their condition and illness _____

Confidence that you can obtain the resources of an interpreter when it is needed _____

Confidence that you can effectively use a skilled interpreter
_____

Source: Muzumdar, J. M., Holiday-Goodman, M., & Black, C. (2010). Cultural competence knowledge and confidence after classroom activities. *American Journal of Pharmaceutical Education, 74*(8), 6.

Based on your responses to the exercises, write a one-paragraph description of yourself as it relates to respect for others.

⫸ Respect for Others and the Emotional Intelligence Framework

Have you ever been in a foreign country or a circumstance where you felt like a complete outsider? What did you want in that circumstance, other than to go home or get out of there?

Self-aware: Examine your attitude toward the people you work with and the patients you treat. Are they cases, revenue, units of production, or independent human beings worthy of your care? Is the focus of your professional aspirations monetary or people?

Self-management: How do you deal with the people you don't like or respect, the patients you have trouble relating to?

Social awareness: The next time you are at work, try to understand what is going on with the people you encounter. What are they really seeking from you, a kind word or a dispassionate clinical opinion?

Relationship management: Try smiling at work one day, and record how it feels. Avoid one negative comment at work, and record how it feels.

⫸ Respect for Others: Personal Learning Plan

These steps can be compiled on a single page containing the following:

What prompted me to develop this plan?

What is the general area for improvement?

What is the specific issue for improvement?

Why is this important to me?

How do I generally act in these areas?

What are my goals?

What prompted this effort?

What strategies are required?

Who/what is necessary to meet my goals with this strategy?

How will I measure the success/failure of this effort?

How long will I focus on this effort?

How will I reflect and capture a lesson from this effort that can be generalized to other circumstances.

⫸ WHAT'S IMPORTANT TO YOU IN THE CHAPTER?

With several of your classmates, discuss the idea/ideas that are most likely to effect a change in your values, attitudes, or behaviors. Be succinct—no more than two sentences.

◈ REFERENCES

American Board of Internal Medicine. (2001). *Project Professionalism*. Philadelphia, PA: Author.

Andersson, L. M., & Pearson, C. M. (1999). Tit for tat? The spiraling effect of incivility in the workplace. *Academy of Management Review, 24*(3), 452–471.

Bartlett II, J. E., & Bartlett, M. E. (2011). Workplace bullying: An integrative literature review. *Advances in Developing Human Resources, 13*(1), 69–84.

Blau, G., & Andersson, L. (2005). Testing a measure of instigated workplace incivility. *Journal of Occupational and Organizational Psychology, 78,* 595–614.

Carnegie, D. (1981). *How to win friends and influence people.* New York, NY: Gallery.

Coyle, J., & Williams, B. (2001). Valuing people as individuals: Development of an instrument through a survey of person-centeredness in secondary care. *Journal of Advanced Nursing, 36,* 450–459.

Maloney, R. J. (2009). *A phenomenological focus on Levinas' concept of alterity interpreted as respect for the other in a healthcare encounter* (Unpublished doctoral dissertation). Widener University, Widener, PA.

Muzumdar, J. M., Holiday-Goodman, M., & Black, C. (2010). Cultural competence knowledge and confidence after classroom activities. *American Journal of Pharmaceutical Education, 74*(8), 1–8.

Peterson, B. (2004). *Cultural intelligence.* Boston, MA: Intercultural Press.

◈ SUGGESTED READINGS

Assemi, M., Cullander, C., & Hudmon, K. S. (2006). Psychometric analysis of a scale assessing self-efficacy for cultural competence in patient counseling. *Annals of Pharmacotherapy, 40,* 2130–2135.

Beach, M. C., Duggan, P. S., Cassell, C. K., & Geller, G. (2007). What does "respect" mean? Exploring the moral obligation of health professionals to respect patients. *Society of General Internal Medicine, 22,* 692–695.

Benditt, T. M. (2008). Why respect matters. *Journal of Value Inquiry, 42,* 487–496.

Earley, P. C., & Mosakowski, E. (2004, October). Cultural intelligence. *Harvard Business Review,* 139–146.

Felblinger, D. M. (2008). Incivility and bullying in the workplace and nurses' shame responses. *Journal of Obstetric, Gynecologic, and Neonatal Nursing, 37,* 234–242.

Forni, P. M. (2008). *The civility solution.* New York, NY: St. Martin's Press.

Langdon, S. W. (2007). Conceptualizations of respect: Qualitative and quantitative evidence of four (five) themes. *Journal of Psychology, 141*(5), 469–484.

McCance, T., Slater, P., & McCormack, B. (2008). Using the caring dimensions inventory as an indicator of person-centeredness nursing. *Journal of Clinical Nursing, 18,* 409–417.

15

The Dark Side

Pre-Assessment: The Dark Side

Mind Mapping

Consider the term below. Without thinking or editing, write down the ideas, concepts, examples, contradictions, and theories that come to mind. Do not array them in any systematic or orderly manner. Scatter them about the page. Now, draw lines between your additions, indicating that there is a relationship between the terms. If something causes something else, indicate this with an arrow. Relationships may be reciprocal—both cause each other—requiring arrows at both ends. Indicate the strength of the relationship by darkening and thickening the lines—stronger relationships have darker and thicker lines. Most important: There is no right answer. Do not compare with your classmates. *What you have is a mind map, your mental representation of the topic. Review to determine if anything has changed following this section.*

Evil

⚙ DESIRED EDUCATIONAL OUTCOMES

- Discuss whether the dark side of professionalism is a continuous variable.
- Describe the personality traits described as the dark triad.

⚙ DESIRED PERSONAL OUTCOME

- Achieve an enhanced ability to recognize nonprofessional behaviors.

Professional status confers unusual power and autonomy on individuals within the practice of that profession. That power and autonomy can be abused. Seven behaviors—when exhibited—diminish individual professionalism, compromise care, weaken the healthcare system, and erode patient trust and confidence. Those seven behaviors, when bundled together, can be termed the dark side of professionalism. The seven behaviors are (American Board of Internal Medicine, 2001):

- *Abuse of power:* Society confers power upon professionals and typically abides by the recommendations of that person. If this power is used for reasons other than the betterment of the patient and society, typically for personal gain, then abuse occurs. Abuse of power can occur in relationships with patients and colleagues. This abuse manifests itself in bias, sexual harassment, and breaches in confidentiality.

- *Arrogance:* Arrogance is an offensive display of superiority and self-importance resulting in haughtiness, vanity, insolence, and disdain.

- *Greed:* Greed predominates when money becomes the driving force. Greed is an inordinate pursuit of power, fame, and money.

- *Misrepresentation:* Misrepresentation is lying and fraud. Lying is consciously failing to tell the truth. Fraud is a conscious misrepresentation of fact intended to mislead.

- *Impairment:* Impairment occurs as a result of alcohol, drugs, or mental impairment.

- *Lack of conscientiousness:* Lack of conscientiousness is the failure to fulfill responsibilities.

- *Conflict of interest:* Situations where the interest of the pharmacist is placed above the patient are conflicts of interest.

Is the Dark Side a Dichotomous Variable?

A DICHOTOMOUS VARIABLE IS AN EITHER/OR proposition. In most circumstances, one is either male or female. With rare exceptions, no person is either completely evil or completely good. Most of us are mosaics of both traits, good at some things and not others; improving on some things and regressing on others; molded by circumstance and blown by the winds of convenience and expediency. No pharmacist is likely to be characterized as completely nonprofessional. A pharmacist who is defrauding Medicare may still be loved by her patients for her empathy and willingness to serve. The dark side, then, is not a dichotomous variable, but a continuous variable that registers degrees of nonprofessional behaviors and traits.

In short, the dark side of professional behavior is simply an expression of inherent personality traits termed the "dark triad." The dark triad represents a social engagement strategy based on exploitation. Each personality trait involves a high degree of selfishness and elevating one's personal needs over the needs of others. Because these traits are not socially desirable, individuals often try to hide them. Along with this external deception, there is often a high level of internal deception regarding these traits as individuals rationalize to themselves why they must engage in this pattern.

How Do You Explain These Behaviors?

THE DARK SIDE OF PROFESSIONALISM can be explained from multiple perspectives. Each offers insight into these behaviors. As with all explanations for human behavior, each of these insights is limited in some manner. Taken together, they give a reasonable explanation for this pattern of professional behavior.

- These behaviors may arise as a function of the impact of cultural norms and the economic system. A consumer focus and a ruthless social Darwinism, unfettered by perspective, may lead to a disregard for others and a sense that "I have to get mine."

- An unconscious need felt as a constant hunger, a feeling of being alone and of being empty, may lead to selfish gratification and a ruthless pursuit of money and power.

Box 15.1 What Personality Traits Explain This Aspect of Professionalism?

The dark side of professionalism can be linked to personality—specifically, three personality traits termed the "dark triad":

❑ *Machiavellianism:* Machiavellianism rests on the following values: a belief in the effectiveness of manipulative tactics for personal gain, a cynical view of human nature, and a moral outlook that elevates expediency over principle. Machiavellians are more likely to make ethically suspect decisions. They are more likely to cheat, lie, and betray others, but do not typically engage in extreme forms of negative behavior.

❑ *Narcissism:* Narcissism is characterized by an inflated view of the self and fantasies of control, admiration, and success. Most individuals possess some level of this trait. At the extremes these traits become problematic. Narcissists may appear arrogant, self-promoting, and less likeable. When publicly censored or challenged, narcissists may react aggressively. At the extreme, narcissism is considered a clinical disorder, rather than a personality trait.

❑ *Psychopathy:* Psychopathy is characterized by a lack of concern for others and the rules of society. A lack of guilt is associated with this trait. These people are characterized by likeability, glibness, and charm, though they are callous, emotionally cold, and unsentimental. They often engage in parasitic lifestyles and utilize criminal behaviors to achieve their ends. They are associated with academic cheating. Like narcissism, at the extreme, psychopathy is a clinical disorder rather than a personality trait.

Source: Adapted from O'Boyle, E. H., Forsyth, D. R., Banks, G. C., & McDaniel, M. A. (2011, October 24). A meta-analysis of the dark triad and work behavior: A social exchange perspective. *Journal of Applied Psychology*, 2.

- Schemas are theories of the self, others, and the world that serve as a cognitive framework for behavior. In other words, what is believed about the self, others, and the world drives behaviors. Inappropriate schemas reflecting abandonment, entitlement, specialness, omnipotence, perfectionism, never being satisfied, and so on provide templates for justifying ruthless professional actions.

- From an evolutionary perspective, behaviors have been selected for their impact on species survival and then transmitted to subsequent generations. In appropriate doses, the behavioral patterns of the dark triad can be presumed to enhance survival for the individual. In short, there is a genetic basis for the behaviors of the dark triad.

- These behaviors may simply be learned. Association with respected mentors who exhibit these behaviors may lead a novice professional to assume that these are the rules of the game for getting ahead.

- Like all behaviors, their variation can be arrayed along a bell curve. People who exhibit the dark triad are simply those at the tail of a normal distribution anchored by good at one tail and evil at the other. Deficiencies in the brain chemistry and circuitry may account for the nonprofessional behaviors. At least 10 interconnected brain regions are involved in an empathy circuit. It is deficiencies in these regions that explain this distribution.

- Parenting that was neglectful or abusive may lie at the root of the nonprofessional behaviors.

Box 15.2   Why Do People Lie?

Lying is not the exception in human behavior. Lying is often spontaneous and unconscious, devoid of cynicism. The reasons people lie include:

- ❑ People lie because they like to, because they derive pleasure from it and a sense of power.
- ❑ People lie to gain an advantage.
- ❑ People lie to achieve an end result.
- ❑ People lie because it is socially advantageous to them, to enhance social prestige.
- ❑ People lie as a means of self-preservation, beginning with a white lie and spreading to a complex web of deceit.

❑   People lie to avoid punishment.

❑   People lie because deception is required to function in daily life.

❑   People lie because the truth may be hurtful, difficult, or painful.

❑   Excessive lying may be a warning sign and plea for help.

❑   People lie to protect their innermost thoughts and feelings.

Source: Adapted from Williams, K. C., Hernandez, E. H., Petrosky, A. R., & Page, R. A. (2009, Winter). The business of lying. *Journal of Leadership, Accountability, and Ethics*, 1–20.

The interesting question is why someone who has economic security, status, and power as a result of their professional licensure would feel the need to risk those things by violating the standards of the profession?

Only the extremely naïve would discount the value of relatively harmless lies that smooth out and maintain the social fabric. Lies that significantly favor one party at the expense of another are a different matter. A professional who "shades" their advice and recommendations to unduly profit and compromise another is clearly outside this realm of lies as social lubrication. A lie told to a child about to undergo an uncomfortable round of chemotherapy is an act of professional kindness; a lie regarding a fatal mistake to protect a license is not.

The Impaired Pharmacist

PROFESSIONALS MAY BE IMPAIRED COGNITIVELY, emotionally, or as a result of substance abuse. Each of these impairments has its own specific cause and is beyond the scope of this book. Generally, larger organizations have formal programs and policies that deal with this matter, particularly related to substance abuse. Programs for cognitive and emotional impairment are not as common. The ideal circumstance is that the professional him- or herself recognizes the impairment, and self-reports the problem, and enters treatment. Typically, discovery of impairment by the company results in a punitive response by the company. Being aware of an impaired colleague, pharmacists have to balance the right of the individual practitioner to privacy with the health and safety of the patients and the integrity of the healthcare system. It is no small thing to report an impaired pharmacist because livelihoods, careers, reputations, and families are at stake.

What is the dark side on this issue? A pharmacist who is aware of his or her impairment and knows that patients are at risk and continues to practice is drifting toward the dark side. They are consciously placing their patients at risk. A pharmacist suffering from situational depression because a child has just died and who tries to soldier on, unaware that their ability to focus is not as sharp as it could be, is something else.

How to Deal with Dark Side Professionals

IT IS NOT LIKELY AS a student that you will knowingly encounter this type of professional. The key here is *knowingly*. It is not likely you will have sufficient encounters to pick up on this trait. As a new graduate, however, you may have to deal with this type of practitioner. A few reminders are in order. They are:

- Practitioners demonstrating this behavior pattern are likely to be very good at it. They are likely to be very subtle in their methods. Only the most egregious examples get noted, and if it is noticed infrequently, it may be explained by others as an aberration.

- Dark side practitioners see others as playing specific roles in their internal psychopathic drama. Specifically, they see themselves as special whereas others are pawns, patrons, patsies, and police. They have the inability to be modest, to accept blame, to act predictably, to react calmly, and to act without aggression. Their goal will be to sabotage your career.

- Be cautious in labeling someone a psychopath. Although several psychopathic tendencies may be evident, only strong evidence should support this designation.

- Greater personal insight reveals personal vulnerabilities and weaknesses that dark side practitioners may prey on. Understand which of your buttons a psychopath might push. The desire to want to "save" someone else should be a red flag. Psychopaths will draw you in and try to establish a personal bond, to your detriment and to their benefit.

- If you believe you are dealing with a psychopathic boss or coworker, document your encounters and their behaviors for your file. These people will be adept at sullying your reputation, so documentation with dates, times, and contemporaneous summaries of conversations will support your claims.

- If changing the situation is impossible, then the best option is to leave. But do so under your own terms as much as possible. Be professional. Get on with your life and career. Avoid assuming any guilt for this circumstance. Some circumstances simply can't be overcome.

Box 15.3   The Dark Side in Action: The Toxic Pharmacist

Robert Courtney was born in 1952 and graduated from pharmacy school in 1975. He was the owner of Research Medical Tower Pharmacy in Kansas City, Missouri. He was described as an "ideal son" and was a deacon in the Assembly of God Church. He was divorced and the father of four children. His patients loved him, describing him as a gentleman who was always fastidiously dressed and groomed. By the time he was 40 years old, Robert owned two pharmacies, drove a Mercedes, lived in one of the most prestigious subdivisions in Kansas City, could afford to buy his second wife a four-carat diamond ring, had pledged $1 million dollars to his church's building fund, was planning to build a 5,000 square foot house, and had amassed $18.7 million in total assets.

Courtney has been described as somewhat aloof, distant, and withdrawn. His moods could shift from ebullience to aloofness. When disagreeing with his second wife about something his face would harden and take on a crazed look like he wanted to murder someone. In public he once yelled at one of his daughters and slapped her at home. He always needed to be in control, even dictating his wife's attire to attend a church event.

In 2002 Courtney pled guilty to 20 federal counts of adulterating and tampering the chemotherapy drugs Taxol and Gemzar. He was sentenced to 30 years in federal prison, was named as defendant in 300 suits for fraud and wrongful death, and was hit with a judgment in the amount of $2.2 billion. From 1990 to 2002, it is estimated that Courtney diluted 98,000 prescriptions for 4,200 patients involving 72 different drugs, including fertility drugs, antibiotics, and drugs to improve blood clotting. Often Courtney dispensed generic drugs when name brands were

(Continues)

Box 15.3   *(Continued)*

called for. In addition to the fraud related to adulterated prescriptions, Courtney had been buying drugs through the gray market, outside the normal channels of distribution.

An Eli Lilly rep first noticed a discrepancy in the amount of Gemzar Courtney was buying and the amount he sold to the doctors in his building. Alerted to this fact, one of the doctors who bought prescriptions from Courtney decided to have them tested. The results indicated that the prescriptions had been diluted from 39% of the called for concentration to almost zero for certain prescriptions. In short, Courtney was dispensing sterile water to patients with terminal and life-threatening conditions.

The question is, How do you explain Courtney's behavior

Source: Adapted from Draper, R. (2003). The toxic pharmacist. *New York Times*, June 8. The complete article is available at http://www.nytimes.com/2003/06/08 /magazine/the-toxic-pharmacist.html and provides a richer description of Courtney. The CNBC television program *American Greed* produced a documentary of this case. It is available at http://www.cnbc.com/id23182570. The program is from season 2, episode 4, and aired on February 27, 2008. Viewing this program is highly recommended. It is powerful in that both Robert Courtney and victims of his acts are presented. At least one of the victims died.

Assignment: What Do the Practitioners/ Others Say?

BE PREPARED TO DISCUSS THE dark side of practice based on any *one* of the following:

- A discussion with your colleagues, or others, on how they feel and what they know about the dark side of practice
- An article on the dark side, either from the research literature or any other source
- A movie/television program/YouTube video about the dark side
- A book on the dark side (literary, historical, psychological, or any other source)

EXERCISES

⫴ Dark Triad

Please complete the questions using the following choices:
SD = strongly disagree; D = disagree; N = neutral; A = agree; SA = strongly agree

1. I tend to manipulate others to get my way. _____
2. I have used deceit or lied to get my way. _____
3. I have used flattery to get my way. _____
4. I tend to exploit others toward my own end. _____
5. I tend to lack remorse. _____
6. I tend to be unconcerned with the morality of my actions. _____
7. I tend to be callous or insensitive. _____
8. I tend to be cynical. _____
9. I tend to want others to admire me. _____
10. I tend to want others to pay attention to me. _____
11. I tend to seek prestige or status. _____
12. I tend to expect special favors from others. _____

Agree and strongly agree responses for questions 1 to 4 indicate a tendency to use Machiavellianism. Agree and strongly agree responses for questions 5 to 8 indicate a tendency to psychopathic behavior. Agree and strongly agree responses for questions 9 to 12 indicate a tendency towards narcissism.

Source: Jonason, P. K., & Webster, G. D. (2010). The dirty dozen: A concise measure of the dark triad. *Psychological Assessment, 22*(2), 429.

⫴ Cheating Behaviors

Please answer yes or no regarding whether you have done any of the following:

1. Paraphrasing material from another source without acknowledging the original author _____

2. Inventing data (e.g., entering nonexistent results into a database) _____

3. Allowing own coursework to be copied by another student _____

4. Fabricating references or a bibliography _____

5. Copying material for coursework from a book or other publication without acknowledging the source _____

6. Altering data (e.g., adjusting data to obtain a significant result) _____

7. Copying another student's coursework with their knowledge _____

8. Ensuring the availability of books or journal articles in the library by deliberately mis-shelving them so other students cannot find them, or by cutting out the relevant article or chapter _____

9. In a situation where students mark each other's work, coming to an agreement with another student or students to mark each other's work more generously than it merits _____

10. Submitting a piece of coursework as an individual piece of work when it has actually been written jointly with another student _____

Calculate your cheating index as the percentage of yes answers to these questions. What does this percentage say about you? Are there implications in this for future practice? Do you consider any of these items not to be cheating?

Source: Newstead, S. E., Franklyn-Stokes, A., & Armstead, P. (1996). Individual differences in student cheating. *Journal of Educational Psychology*, *88*(2), 232.

⊕ Reasons for Cheating or Not Cheating

Please check any items that you believe explain why you would cheat or not cheat.

For cheating

1. To help a friend _____

2. Time pressure _____

3. Extenuating circumstances _____

4. Peer pressure _____

5. To increase the grade _____

6. Monetary reward _____

7. Fear of failure _____

8. Everybody does it _____

9. Laziness _____

For not cheating

1. It would devalue my achievement. _____

2. It is immoral or dishonest. _____

3. Personal pride. _____

4. It was unnecessary or pointless. _____

5. Shame or embarrassment at being caught. _____

6. I never thought of it. _____

7. Fear of detection or punishment. _____

8. I would not know how to go about it. _____

9. It would be unfair to other students. _____

10. Situation did not arise. _____

Compare your responses on this section with several of your classmates'.

Source: Newstead, S. E., Franklyn-Stokes, A., & Armstead, P. (1996). Individual differences in student cheating. *Journal of Educational Psychology*, 88(2), 233.

Based on your responses, write a one-paragraph description of yourself as it relates to the dark side.

⫸ The Dark Side and the Emotional Intelligence Framework

How high is the incidence of cheating in your school? How is it handled?

> *Self-aware:* List instances where you may have violated some aspect of academic integrity. If you have done so, what rationalizations have you

used? If you haven't, how do you explain this? Repeat the same process for lying.

Self-management: Based on your experience, what advice would you give a new student regarding the temptation to cheat?

Social awareness: Pick the person in your class most likely to violate norms of academic integrity. What about them cues you to make this assessment? (Please keep this choice private.)

Relationship management: In dealing with technicians at work, what things would constitute an abuse of power on the part of the pharmacist?

◈ Personal Learning Plan: The Dark Side

These steps can be compiled on a single page containing the following:

What prompted me to develop this plan?

What is the general area for improvement?

What is the specific issue for improvement?

Why is this important to me?

How do I generally act in these areas?

What are my goals?

What prompted this effort?

What strategies are required?

Who/what is necessary to meet my goals with this strategy?

How will I measure the success/failure of this effort?

How long will I focus on this effort?

How will I reflect and capture a lesson from this effort that can be generalized to other circumstances?

⬥ WHAT'S IMPORTANT TO YOU IN THE CHAPTER?

With several of your classmates, discuss the idea/ideas that are most likely to effect a change in your values, attitudes, or behaviors. Be succinct—no more than two sentences.

⬥ REFERENCES

American Board of Internal Medicine. (2001). *Project Professionalism.* Philadelphia, PA: Author.

Draper, R. (2003). The toxic pharmacist. *New York Times*, June 8.

Jonason, P. K., & Webster, G. D. (2010). The dirty dozen: A concise measure of the dark triad. *Psychological Assessment, 22*(2), 420–432.

Newstead, S. E., Franklyn-Stokes, A., & Armstead, P. (1996). Individual differences in student cheating. *Journal of Educational Psychology, 88*(2), 229–241.

O'Boyle, E. H., Forsyth, D. R., Banks, G. C., & McDaniel, M. A. (2011, October 24). A meta-analysis of the dark triad and work behavior: A social exchange perspective. *Journal of Applied Psychology*, 1–23.

Williams, K. C., Hernandez, E. H., Petrosky, A. R., & Page, R. A. (2009, Winter). The business of lying. *Journal of Leadership, Accountability, and Ethics*, 1–20.

⬥ SUGGESTED READINGS

Austin, E. J., Farrelly, D., Black, C., & Moore, H. (2007). Emotional intelligence, Machiavellianism and emotional manipulation: Does EI have a dark side? *Personality and Individual Differences, 43*, 179–189.

Babiak, P., & Hare, R. D. (2006). *Snakes in suits.* New York, NY: Harper Collins.

Baron-Cohen, S. (2011). *The science of evil.* New York, NY: Basic.

Farber, N. J., Gilibert, S. G., Aboff, B. M., Collier, V. U., Weiner, J., & Boyer, G. (2005). Physicians' willingness to report impaired colleagues. *Social Science and Medicine, 61*, 1772–1775.

Gilbert, P. (2002). Evolutionary approaches to psychopathy and cognitive therapy. *Journal of Cognitive Psychotherapy, 16*(3), 263–294.

Kenna, G. A., Erickson, C., & Tommasello, A. (2006). Understanding substance abuse and dependence by the pharmacy profession. *U.S. Pharmacist, 5*, 21–33.

Leahy, R. L. (1992). Cognitive therapy on Wall Street: Schemas and scripts of invulnerability. *Journal of Cognitive Psychotherapy, 6*(4), 245–258.

Lubit, R. H. (2004). *Coping with toxic managers, subordinates . . . and other difficult people.* Upper Saddle River, NJ: FT Press.

Maher, B. A., & Maher, W. B. (1994). Personality and psychopathology: A historical perspective. *Journal of Abnormal Psychology, 103*(1), 72–77.

Nikelly, A. (2006). The pathogenesis of greed: Causes and consequences. *International Journal of Applied Psychoanalytic Studies, 3*(1), 65–78.

Rabi, S. M., Patton, L. R., Fjortoft, N., & Zgarrick, D. P. (2006) Characteristics, prevalence, attitudes, and perceptions of academic dishonesty among pharmacy students. *American Journal of Pharmacy Education, 70*(4), 1–8.

Reimann, M., & Zimbardo, P. G. The dark side of social encounters: Prospects for a neuroscience of human evil. *Journal of Neuroscience, Psychology, and Economics, 4*(3), 174–180.

Saulsberry, M. D., Brown III, U. J., Heyliger, S. O., Beale, R. L. (2011). Effect of dispositional traits on pharmacy students' attitude toward cheating. *American Journal of Pharmaceutical Education, 75*(4), 1–8.

Waska, R. (2004). Greed and the frightening rumble of psychic hunger. *American Journal of Psychoanalysis, 64*(3), 253–266.

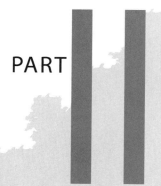

PART II

Summary: Commandments for Professionalism

At the end of each chapter you were asked to list what was important to you in that chapter. Collect the statements for each chapter and review. Can any statements be combined, eliminated, or synthesized into simpler and more personally useful statements? The task is to arrive at the fewest statements that capture the essence of what is important and memorable. In other words, what are you likely to remember in 6 months or a year? Consult with your classmates on this exercise.

⫸ WHAT'S IMPORTANT TO YOU IN THE CHAPTER?

Professionalism:

Altruism:

Accountability:

Duty, Honor, and Integrity:

Excellence:

Respect for Others:

The Dark Side:

PART III

Clinical Responsibility

The school's obligation is to provide you the clinical information to make lives better. Not knowing a dose, missing a side effect, or utilizing poor technique can impact a patient. Clinical responsibility is not just about being technically adept, however. It is also about understanding how you think and make decisions; about how you deal with success and failure; about how you react to and cope with errors; about how you keep your personal and professional life in balance; about how you relate to and interact with other professionals; and about how you deal with stress and burnout.

Your obligation is to understand how you operate as a person, as a clinician, and as a professional. Your clinical responsibility is to understand you, because you are the instrument that delivers the clinical expertise. This self-awareness, this self-management is your duty; it is your commitment to excellence.

CHAPTER 16

Expertise and Thinking

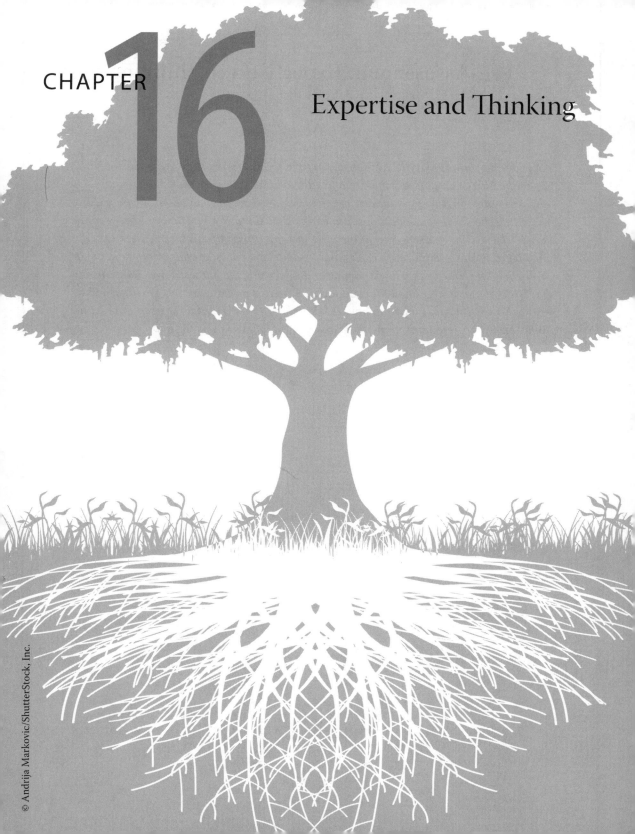

Pre-Assessment: Expertise and Thinking

Mind Mapping

Consider the terms arrayed on the page. For each term, without thinking or editing, write down the ideas, concepts, examples, contradictions, and theories that come to mind. Do not array them in any systematic or orderly manner. Scatter them about the page. Now, draw lines between your additions, indicating that there is a relationship between the terms. If something causes something else, indicate this with an arrow. Relationships may be reciprocal—both cause each other—requiring arrows at both ends. Indicate the strength of the relationship by darkening and thickening the lines; stronger relationships have darker and thicker lines. Most important: There is no right answer. Do not compare with your classmates. *What you have is a mind map, your mental representation of the topic. Review to determine if anything has changed following this section.*

Intuition
Judgment
Wisdom
Stupidity

⫸ DESIRED EDUCATIONAL OUTCOMES

- Describe what separates the expert from the novice.
- Define practical intelligence.
- List the devices that aid in thinking.

⫸ DESIRED PERSONAL OUTCOME

- Achieve an enhanced ability to think.

What Is Expertise? Who Is an Expert?

A PROFESSIONAL SCHOOL IS A DELIBERATE attempt to create an expert. Expertise is domain specific; that is, what is required of an expert trial attorney is different from the requirements of an expert Doctor of Pharmacy, which is different from the requirements of an expert psychotherapist. Expertise can be shown in skills, knowledge, or abilities; in processes such as decision making; or in output such as a decision. An expert is someone who demonstrates expertise. Cognitively, experts possess extensive and up-to-date content knowledge, highly developed perceptual abilities, a sense of what is relevant, an ability to simplify complex problems, and an ability to adapt to exceptions. They can perceive meaningful patterns in large masses of information, are faster, have superior long-term and short-term memories, see problems at a deeper level, can anticipate, have a global view of the situation, and have a rich repertoire of strategies.

What Are the Stages of Expertise?

THE VIEW TAKEN IN THIS text is that expertise is a developmental process. People are not born experts; they develop into experts. The development of expertise goes through stages. The Model of Domain Learning (MDL) posits three stages in expertise development. Acclimation is the initial stage. In this stage learners orient (acclimate) themselves to a complex and unfamiliar domain. The learner has limited and fragmented knowledge of the domain. The next stage is competence, in which the learner demonstrates foundational knowledge that is cohesive and principled in structure. Typical domain-specific problems become familiar and the learner demonstrates both surface-level and deep-level strategies. In the final stage of proficiency and expertise, the knowledge base is both wide and deep. Experts engage in problem finding and contribute to new knowledge in the domain.

The Guild model posits seven stages for expert development. The seven stages are as follows (adapted from Hoffman, Shadbolt, Burton, & Klein, 1995):

- *Naivette:* One who is totally ignorant of the domain.

- *Novice:* Someone who is new—a probationary member. There has been some, minimal exposure to the domain.

- *Initiate:* Someone who has been through an initiation ceremony—a novice who has begun introductory instruction.

- *Apprentice:* Someone who is learning—a student undergoing a program of instruction beyond the introductory level. The length of the apprenticeship depends on the domain, ranging from about 1 to 12 years.

- *Journeyman:* A person who can perform a day's labor unsupervised, although working under orders. An experienced and reliable worker, or one who has achieved a level of competence. It is possible to remain at this level for life.

- *Expert:* The distinguished or brilliant journeyman, highly regarded by peers, whose judgments are uncommonly accurate and reliable, and whose performance shows consummate skills or knowledge derived from extensive experience with subdomains.

- *Master:* Traditionally, a master is a journeyman or expert who is qualified to teach those at a lower level; also one of an elite group of experts whose judgments set the regulations, standards, or ideals. A master also can be an expert who is regarded by others as being "the" expert, or the "real" expert, especially with regard to subdomain knowledge.

Pharmacists: Experts at What?

Pharmacists have two primary functions: one is clinical and the other is distributive. This chapter mainly deals with pharmacist expertise in the clinical role.

Clinical Expertise

An *A* grade on a case study or a round of applause following a case presentation is one thing. These situations are great training, but do not reflect the reality of practice. Pharmacy clinicians deal with the following (adapted from Patel, Kaufman, & Magder, 1996):

- *Ill-structured problems:* Real problems are seldom clean. Sometimes it is not clear there is a problem until later. Choices are not laid out for examination. Clinical problems have not been sanitized as they are in the classroom to highlight a teaching point.

- *Uncertain and dynamic environments:* The real world is ambiguous, with incomplete information embedded in environments that may change with time.

- *Competing, ill-defined, or shifting goals:* Conflicts, tradeoffs, and shifting priorities are the order of the day.

- *Action-feedback loops:* Cause and effect are hard to discern. Was the outcome a function of the clinical choices made, a residual from the original condition, or a random or idiosyncratic response?

- *Time stress and high risk:* Decisions need to be made on the fly, while tired or distracted where there is no margin for error.

- *Multiple players:* Clinical choices often have to account for multiple actors with different responsibilities and objectives.

Clinical problems are not multiple choice tests. They are not even essay tests. They are an oral exam where you don't really know what the examiners are looking for and you don't know how long it is going to last, or even when it will start. You don't know if they want the short answer or a detailed explanation. And you won't be able to tell how you are doing by their facial expressions, because they will be sitting behind a screen. All you know is if you don't pass, you don't graduate. Clinical problems are the ultimate high stakes exam; the NAPLEX pales in comparison.

What Do Experts Do That a Novice Can't?

COMPARED TO A NOVICE, EXPERTS perceive patterns and opportunities in what appears to the novice to be incoherent information; the expert sees data, the novice sees noise. Experts are faster at processing information and utilizing the appropriate skill; they have superior long-term and short-term memory; see problems at a deeper, more principled layer than the novice; and spend more time assessing the problem prior to solving it.

How Do Experts Think?

CLINICAL EXPERTISE IS ORGANIZED INTO four levels. At the first level observations are made that are recognized as being potentially relevant to solving the problem. Some of these observations are then recognized and declared to have clinical significance and are termed *findings*. This is the second level. Findings are then grouped into clusters that begin to suggest a prediagnostic interpretation of the problem. These clusters, the third level of expertise, are termed *facets*, from which interim hypotheses are formed. Another way to think of facets is that they are the equivalent of mental blueprints stored in long-term memory as a result of prior experiences that serve to facilitate, simplify, and expedite the thinking process. Sometimes they are termed *illness scripts*. At the same time, clinicians are accessing scripts, based on experience, for various types of patients. Expert clinicians merge their scripts for a particular disease profile with their scripts for a particular type of patient. A diagnosis, the fourth level, results from the overlap of these scripts.

The key feature of this process is the idea of a pretested and preloaded script, or mental blueprint. Because of this, the expert clinician does not have to stop and consciously work through the process, step by step, nor consciously recall or consult basic biomedical principles that underlie the process. Experience tells them this is what it is and what will work without

Box 16.1   What Do We Know About Experts and Expertise?

Experts and expertise have been studied extensively in numerous areas including sports, medicine, music, chess, the military, and leadership. Here is what we know about experts and expertise.

- ❑ Expertise requires practice, years of practice. For some disciplines an acceptable level of performance may be achieved relatively easily or quickly—months to a few years. High-level expertise generally takes at least a decade.
- ❑ Expertise is domain specific. Being expert at oncology does not qualify one as an expert in pediatrics. Watch Hall of Fame basketball player Charles Barkley swing a golf club to understand this point. Experts outside their realm of expertise solve problems as a novice would.
- ❑ Expertise requires deliberate practice. Deliberate practice is specifically tailored to enhance a skill.
- ❑ Experts and novices see the world with different eyes. A world class conductor looks at a musical score differently than does a novice.
- ❑ Expertise may blind to other approaches and points of view.
- ❑ Expertise can be either routine or adaptive. Routine experts solve the typical problems for the domain. Adaptive expertise solves the novel problem.
- ❑ Some challenging problems are too large for a single perspective; they require multiple experts for resolution.

Source: Adapted from Clark, R. C. (2008). *Building expertise*. San Francisco, CA: Pfeiffer, 7.

consciously remembering the details of why it is this and why this works. Consider never having been in a major city and having to locate a destination. Even with a map or a GPS system you will likely look for and double check the street signs and drive cautiously to avoid missing a turn. You may even slow down to admire the architecture and ruminate on the nuances of how the city is laid out. You are going to get there, eventually. A real problem arises if traffic patterns are disrupted due to construction that is not reflected on the map or in the GPS system. In contrast, someone who drives this route every day will likely be more or less on autopilot, knowing where the bottlenecks are and paying attention to only a few critical turns and merges. Having driven the route daily, the city's architecture no longer attracts unless it is significantly altered. Even unanticipated bottlenecks are easily negotiated because several alternative routes are known. The experienced driver gets there as quickly and as easily as possible.

A first-year practitioner should have a relatively functional set of scripts for specific diseases and specific types of patients. These scripts only improve if the practitioner takes the time and makes the effort to examine their choices against the outcomes those choices produced. Experience then shapes and polishes those scripts as the practitioner moves through their career. Refusing to or neglecting to examine these discrepancies waylays the progression towards expertise. Time on the job is not the answer; time on the job coupled with reflection and continuous learning is the vehicle.

Clinical Thinking and Clinical Decisions

THE FOUNDATION FOR EFFECTIVE CLINICAL decision making is evidence. The quality and availability of that evidence are critical. Implicit in this reliance is the idea that clinical decision making is completely rational, that it is scientific. Unfortunately, human beings do not make decisions in a completely scientific and rational manner. The human brain did not evolve as an organ to calculate probabilities or make statistical inferences. The human brain evolved as an organ for survival. Human thinking and decision making are subject to well-known biases and traps. Examples of these include (adapted from Hammond, Keeney, & Raiffa, 2006):

- *The anchoring trap:* The human mind inordinately focuses on the first impressions, information, and data that it receives. Subsequent decisions are then anchored to this initial impression. Anchors include comments by a colleague, a statistic in an article, stereotypes about people, and historical trends or events. If the first clinical recommendation you make results in an idiosyncratic reaction, in subsequent recommendations you will always factor in this consequence, whether appropriate or not.

- *The status-quo trap:* Humans display a strong bias for things as they are. To make a change incurs personal responsibility and the possibility of criticism and derision. Following an accepted protocol protects the clinician from rebuke and liability. The problem is that protocols become outdated, may not apply to this patient, or may be only marginally effective.

- *The sunk-cost trap:* The sunk-cost trap involves continuing to pursue a course of action that you recommended even though that course of action is not working. It is the idea of throwing good money after bad. The sunk-cost trap is persistence taken to an illogical and ineffective conclusion.

- *The confirming evidence trap:* In making decisions, humans have a tendency to look for information that confirms their point of view or predetermined choice. Information that does not support our point of view is discounted.

- *The framing trap:* How a decision choice is framed significantly impacts the choices made. Choices framed as a gain rather than a loss will impact the decision. Saying a drug has a 90 percent success rate begets one decision. Saying it has a 1 in a 1,000 chance for a fatal brain infection may beget a different decision.

- *The overconfidence trap:* Most of us overrate out abilities. We all tend to believe we are above average.

- *The prudence trap:* We adjust our best estimate to include a "fudge" factor just to be safe. If we believe a 10-day course of treatment is correct we will recommend 12 days just to be certain.

- *The recallability trap:* Anything that distorts or enhances your ability to recall information in a balanced way will bias future choices. A fatal error with a patient will never be forgotten and will likely impact your clinical decisions for a lifetime.

The point is to recognize and understand that you as a clinician are making decisions that may be less than optimal because, like all humans, your thinking is flawed. The only defense against these biases is to be aware of them and to test and retest your choices with rigor and discipline.

Are There Different Types of Thinking?

ANALYTICAL THINKING IS DELIBERATE AND conscious. We know we are doing it and can describe how we do it. Working through a case in order to make a recommendation based on the observable, concrete physical and clinical evidence is an example of analytical thinking. It is the process of being scientific and rational. In contrast, thinking that is unconscious and rapid is intuitive. We cannot describe how we do this type of thinking; it just happens. Recommendations that begin with "I have a feeling" are examples of intuitive thinking. This section focuses on intuition, judgment, and wisdom as examples of intuitive thinking.

What Is Intuition?

Intuition is the "affectively charged judgments that arise through rapid, non-conscious, and holistic associations" (Dane & Pratt, 2009, p. 4). In contrast, the conscious processing of problems is deliberate, rational, and sequential. Intuition has a role in how problems are solved, as an input to moral decisions, and as an aid in creativity where multiple elements are fused in a creative synthesis. Intuition is often described as a gut feeling, instinct, common sense, or a premonition. Much high-level thinking is intuitive, operating like the autopilot in a jet liner without conscious involvement or attention. The fictional character Sherlock Holmes described how he solved a problem as, "From long habit the train of thoughts ran so swiftly through my mind that I arrived at the conclusion without consciousness of the intermediate steps" (Greenhalgh, 2002, p. 396). Intuition involves pattern recognition, similarity recognition, commonsense understanding, and a sense of salience. In a clinical context, involvement with the patient and their care aids in intuition.

Intuition is neither inferior nor superior to other modes of thinking. It is, however, likely to be more effective in certain instances, such as when the decision maker is more experienced and confident; for tasks that involve judgments with no objective criteria but have political, ethical, esthetic, or behavioral overtones; and when time is short.

What Is Wisdom?

Wisdom is an elusive concept of interest to humans since antiquity. Wisdom may be defined as ". . . the application of tacit knowledge as mediated by values toward the goal of achieving a common good . . . through a balance among multiple intrapersonal, interpersonal, and extrapersonal interests . . ." (Sternberg, 1998, p. 353). The key aspect of this definition is the idea of balancing competing interests. An alternative definition of wisdom is "expertise in the fundamental pragmatics of life" (Baltes & Staudinger, 2000, p. 124). This definition rests on the idea of an understanding of the essence of the human condition and the conduct of a good life. The following criteria outline the nature of wisdom (adapted from Baltes & Staudinger, 2000):

- Wisdom addresses important and difficult questions and strategies about conduct and the meaning of life.

- Wisdom includes knowing about the limits of knowledge and the uncertainties of the world.

- Wisdom represents a truly superior level of knowledge, judgment, and advice.

- Wisdom constitutes knowledge with extraordinary scope, depth, measure, and balance.

- Wisdom involves a perfect synergy of mind and character, that is, an orchestration of knowledge and virtues.

- Wisdom represents knowledge used for the good or well-being of oneself and of others.

- Wisdom is easily recognized when manifested, although difficult to achieve and to specify.

Those who are wise have a rich factual knowledge about life, a rich procedural knowledge about life, an understanding of the issues related to each stage of life, an understanding of life's priorities and what is valuable, and an understanding that life is uncertain. Wisdom is the art of living a life that is beneficial to oneself, others, and society at large. Wisdom is an understanding of what is important.

What Is Judgment?

Judgment is the ability to "infer, estimate, and predict the character of unknown events" (Hastie & Dawes, 2001, p. 48). Judgment is the thinking process used when you don't have all the information. Imagine trying to predict the true biological age of a patient based on only the visibly apparent cues. Hair color, body movement, skin tone and texture, clothes, voice, and the like are all cues that are used to make this judgment. From these cues the age of the patient is inferred, estimated, and predicted. In a clinical context, a significant literature may exist on a disease state along with a significant literature on a drug. As long as the patient fits the accepted profile on which this information is based, a clinical decision is straightforward. However, if a particular patient is outside this known profile (morbidly obese, an unusual comorbidity, etc.), then a therapeutic choice and outcome can only be inferred or estimated. Beginning a recommendation with a phrase such as, "My best guess" is an indicator of judgment.

What Is Practical Intelligence?

A perfect diagnosis coupled with a perfect medication therapy protocol is useless if it can't be implemented or achieved. Practical intelligence is the pragmatic know-how to get things done. The ideal protocol is one thing; the practical protocol, in that it is feasible, is another. The former is a theory; the latter is a plan. The know-how to get things done is based on the acquisition of the complex rules of how the organization and people work in a specific context. Generally, these rules are not openly expressed or explicitly taught. It is up to the individual to read the subtle cues and make the appropriate inferences. Learning in this fashion is termed *tacit learning* and is the foundation of practical intelligence. The ease with which one acquires this practical know-how is a measure of one's practical intelligence. A clinician lacking in the practical knowledge to get things done cannot be considered an expert. The practical knowledge of how drugs flow through the system, which departments and personalities facilitate or impede this flow, how the drugs get paid for, and how adherent the patient is likely to be is embedded and inseparable from any medication therapy program. For the pharmacist, practical intelligence regarding the distribution function and mastery of that process is inherent in the journey to expertise.

What Is Stupidity?

THIS IS A CHAPTER ABOUT thinking. Stupidity is the result of not thinking. It is not a measure of intelligence or capability, because truly smart people often do stupid things. Stupidity is a result of thinking becoming frozen. Excessive adherence to rules, protocols, and internal schema in the face of the evidence is stupidity. Stupidity is the "learned corruption of learning" (Welles, 1991, p. 1). Stupidity is the "unquestioning acceptance of any one set of constraints or axioms that algorithmically 'determine' the problem-solving steps one needs to take in order to produce the desired behavior" (Moldoveanu & Langer, 2002, p. 229) An effective technique for dealing with stupidity is to ask yourself: Why are we doing it this way? If the answer is because we have always done it this way, rather than because it produces the best results, then caution is in order. Chico Marx in the movie *Duck Soup* captured this idea when he said, "Who are you going to believe, me or your own eyes." It is the objective evidence that determines whether a decision is correct. It is not the rote adherence to protocol.

Expertise at Work

THE FOLLOWING IS A SAMPLE scenario related to expertise involving RPG (recent pharmacy graduate):

RPG hated to see a new order for a TPN solution come down. It took him so long to do the calculations. The number of variables to be considered was daunting. The last time he worked on a TPN the rest of the staff seemed to be sending subtle cues that he was taking too long. To get it right RPG had to grind the calculations. He had to stop and think at each stage, calculate, and recalculate. Generally, he had to go back and start over because he had missed a critical fact and the result wouldn't work. Something would be missing, not in the right dose, an incompatibility emerged, or the volume was off. His worksheet was a confusing mess. When starting the calculations, RPG felt for a moment the panic of sitting down to a test in school and not knowing how to do the problem.

RPG noticed that one of his colleagues didn't seem to have any problems with TPN solutions. RPG asked if he could look at her worksheets.

They were clean and methodical, and there was a logical progression to the calculations. There were far fewer steps on these sheets than on his. RPG wanted to ask this colleague how she did it.

How would you recommend RPG handle the situation?

Practical Intelligence at Work

THE FOLLOWING IS A SAMPLE scenario related to practical intelligence involving RPG (recent pharmacy graduate):

> RPG considered the invitation to join the P and T committee an honor. She understood the critical role the committee played in drug therapy for the institutions. At the end of the first meeting she was not sure that her comments had been well received by the members of the committee, particularly the one that challenged the interpretation of the results of one of the studies being cited. The committee chair had quickly moved the discussion along following this comment and paid little attention to it. It seemed that the other members of the committee either looked away or glared as she was contributing. RPG was left to ponder what this meant about the committee.

How would you recommend RPG handle the situation?

Assignment: What Do the Practitioners/ Others Say?

BE PREPARED TO DISCUSS EXPERTISE and thinking based on any *one* of the following:

- A discussion with your colleagues, or others, on how they feel and what they know about expertise and thinking
- An article on expertise and thinking, either from the research literature or any other source
- A movie/television program/YouTube video about expertise and thinking
- A book on expertise and thinking (literary, historical, psychological, or any other source).

EXERCISES

1. Relate the "Guild" model of expertise development to the stages of a pharmacist's education and career.

2. With your classmates, discuss what an expert pharmacy clinician should be able to do. List at least three attributes.

Case Analysis

A clinical situation is an exercise in case analysis. The time-honored steps in case analysis are as follows:

1. Identify the problem.

2. Assess by collecting history and physical data.

3. Formulate competing hypotheses, diagnoses, alternatives, and so on.

4. Gather additional information and conduct research in support of each hypothesis, diagnosis, alternative, and so on.

5. Select a specific hypothesis, diagnosis, or alternative as correct.

6. Develop a plan of action.

7. Implement and evaluate choice.

Tips on case analysis:

1. Read through the case quickly to get a general impression of the problem. Highlight any points that jump out. Begin to formulate the problem.

2. To focus attention, use the following devices.

    a. *Consider all factors (CAF):* Ask yourself whether all the important factors have been considered.

    b. *Other people's views (OPV):* How would another clinician look at this same problem? Is there an alternative view of the problem?

    c.   *Plus, minus, interesting (PMI):* Which facts support your hypothesis, which facts do not, and which facts are interesting but irrelevant?

  3. In making the decision, use the following aids:

    a.   Clarify what the purpose of the decision is. In working through the choices remain focused on this purpose.

    b.   What are both the short-term and long-term consequences of the choices?

    c.   If I approached the problem from another person's point of view, what would the decision be?

    d.   Is it possible to look at the problem from a different perspective?

    e.   Does the proposed choice violate or support my values?

Source: Adapted from de Bono, E. (1994). *de Bono's thinking course.* New York, NY: Facts on File.

With several of your classmates, use the sequence outlined above to work through a clinical case from one of your other classes.

⫸ Six Hat Thinking

Edward de Bono developed the Six Thinking Hat Method. Trying to do too many things at once when trying to solve a problem results in confusion. With the Six Thinking Hat Method, only one thing is done at a time. The following are the six different types of hats and the thinking they represent (adapted from de Bono, 1999):

> *White hat thinking:* White hat thinking is mimicking the computer. A computer is neutral. It does not interpret, nor offer shades of meaning. It is an instrument that deals in facts and information. White hat thinking is objective, analytical. White hat thinking separates information into tiers, that which is proven and absolutely true and that which is believed to be true, but not yet verified. White hat thinking excludes intuition, hunches, and choices based on experience.

Red hat thinking: Red hat thinking is about emotion and feeling. It is the opposite of white hat thinking. Ultimately, all decisions are emotional. White hat (analytical) thinking provides a thinking map. In the end, our values and emotions determine the route we take. There is no need to justify an emotion; we just feel that way. Red hat thinking accounts for intuition and hunches as well as deep emotions that might color our choices, such as fear, anger, and jealousy, and transient emotions that occur while working through the problem.

Black hat thinking: Black hat thinking is the hat of caution. It is not balanced. It is a conscious attempt to consider everything that might go wrong. Black hat thinking is risk assessment—an assessment of the future consequences of a decision taken. Black hat thinking is the most important hat; it's overuse must be guarded against. It is easier to be negative than to be constructive.

Yellow hat thinking: Yellow hat thinking is the opposite of black hat thinking; it is positive and optimistic without being delusional or being a Pollyanna. Yellow hat thinking is a search for value and benefit in our actions that is grounded in logic and analysis. Yellow hat thinking is about visions and dreams.

Green hat thinking: Green hat thinking is about new ideas, perceptions, change, and creativity. Green hat thinking attempts to go beyond the known and the obvious in pursuit of a new and better way of doing things.

Blue hat thinking: Blue hat thinking is about control, about orchestrating which type of thinking is appropriate at what stage of the process. It is thinking about the type of thinking a problem requires. Blue hat thinking says we have spent enough time examining the negative aspects of this problem, it is now time to examine the benefits to be gained from our choice.

1. With several of your classmates, use the Six Hat Thinking method to work through a clinical case from one of your other classes.

2. By yourself, use the Six Hat Thinking method to work through your plans following graduation.

Based on your responses, write a one-paragraph description of yourself as it relates to expertise and thinking.

⦚⦚ Practical Intelligence and the Emotional Intelligence Framework

Success as a professional demands that we learn things about ourselves, managing others, and managing our careers. The things learned must be practical rather than academic, informal rather than formal, and tacit rather than directly taught.

Self-aware: What do you know about yourself that lets you maximize your daily productivity? How did you learn this?

Self-management: How do you motivate yourself to perform? How did you learn this?

Social awareness: What is the secret at work of gaining the respect of your superiors? Your coworkers? What is the secret at work to getting what you want from your superiors? Your coworkers?

Relationship management: In your personal relationships, how do you reward people when they do something you like or approve of? In your personal relationships, how do you punish people when they do something you don't like or approve of? How did you learn this?

⦚⦚ Personal Learning Plan: Practical Intelligence

These steps can be compiled on a single page containing the following:

What prompted me to develop this plan?

What is the general area for improvement?

What is the specific issue for improvement?

Why is this important to me?

How do I generally act in these areas?

What are my goals?

What prompted this effort?

What strategies are required?

Who/what is necessary to meet my goals with this strategy?

How will I measure the success/failure of this effort?

How long will I focus on this effort?

How will I reflect and capture a lesson from this effort that can be generalized to other circumstances.

⬥ WHAT'S IMPORTANT TO YOU IN THE CHAPTER?

With several of your classmates, discuss the idea/ideas that are most likely to effect change in your values, attitudes, or behaviors. Be succinct—no more than two sentences.

⬥ REFERENCES

Baltes, P. B., & Staudinger, U. M. (2000). Wisdom: A metaheuristic (pragmatic) to orchestrate mind and virtue toward excellence. *American Psychologist, 55*, 122–136.

Clark, R. C. (2008). *Building expertise.* San Francisco, CA: Pfeiffer.

Dane, E., & Pratt, M. G. (2009). Conceptualizing and measuring intuition: A review of recent trends. *International Review of Industrial and Organizational Psychology, 24*, 1–40.

de Bono, E. (1994). *de Bono's thinking course.* New York, NY: Facts on File.

de Bono, E. (1999). *Six thinking hats.* New York, NY: Back Bay.

Greenhalgh, T. (2002). Intuition and evidence—Uneasy bedfellows. *British Journal of General Practice, 52*(478), 394–400.

Hammond, J. S., Keeney, R. L., & Raiffa, H. (2006, January). The hidden traps in decision making. *Harvard Business Review*, 118–126.

Hastie, R., & Dawes, R. M. (2001). *Rational choice in an uncertain world.* Thousand Oaks, CA: Sage.

Hoffman, R. R., Shadbolt, N. R., Burton, A. M., & Klein, G. (1995). Eliciting knowledge from experts: A methodological analysis. *Organizational Behavior and Human Decision Processes, 62*(2), 129–158.

Moldoveanu, M., & Langer, E. (2002). When "stupid" is smarter than we are. In: R. J. Sternber (Ed.), *Why smart people can be so stupid* (pp. 212–231). New Haven, CT: Yale University Press.

Patel, V. L., Kaufman, D. R., & Magder, S. A. (1996). The acquisition of medical expertise in complex dynamic environments. In: K. A. Ericsson (Ed.), *The road to excellence* (pp. 127–165). Mahwah, NJ: Lawrence Erlbaum.

Sternberg, R. (1998). A balance theory of wisdom. *Review of General Psychology, 2*(4), 347–365.

Welles, J. F. (1991). *The story of stupidity*. Orient, NY: Mount Pleasant Press.

⊹ SUGGESTED READINGS

Albrecht, S. (2009). Evidence-based medicine in pharmacy practice. *US Pharmacist, 34*(10), 14–18.

Alexander, P. A. (2003). The development of expertise: The journey from acclimation to proficiency. *Educational Researcher, 32*(8), 10–14.

Ardelt, M. (2004). Wisdom as expert knowledge system: A critical review of a contemporary operationalization of an ancient concept. *Human Development, 47,* 257–285.

Bornstein, B. H., & Emler, A. C. (2001). Rationality in medical decision making: A review of the literature on doctors' decision-making biases. *Journal of Evaluation in Clinical Practice, 7*(2), 97–107.

Ericsson, K. A., & Charness, N. (1994). Expert performance. *American Psychologist, 49*(8), 725–747.

Ericsson, K. A., Charness, N., Feltovich, P. J., & Hoffman, R. R. (2006). *The Cambridge handbook of expertise and expert performance*. Cambridge, UK: Cambridge University Press.

Ericsson, K. A., Whyte, J., & Ward, P. (2007). Expert performance in nursing. *Advances in Nursing Science, 30*(1), 58–71.

Farrington-Darby, T., & Wilson, J. R. (2006) The nature of expertise: A review. *Applied Ergonomics, 37,* 17–32.

Fox, C. (1997). A confirmatory factor analysis of the structure of tacit knowledge in nursing. *Journal of Nursing Education, 36*(10), 459–466.

King, L., & Appleton, J. V. (1997). Intuition: A critical review of the research and rhetoric. *Journal of Advanced Nursing, 26,* 194–202.

Mockler, R. J., & Dologite, D. G. (1999). Learning how to learn: Nurturing professional growth through cognitive mapping. *New England Journal of Entrepreneurship, 2*(2), 65–80.

Nagelkerk, J. (2001). *Diagnostic reasoning.* Philadelphia, PA: Saunders.

Patel, V. L., Arocha, J. F., & Kaufman, D. R. (1999). Expertise and tacit knowledge in medicine. In: R. J. Sternberg & J. A. Horvath (Eds.), *Tacit knowledge in professional practice* (pp. 75–99). New York, NY: Routledge.

Quirk, M. (2006). *Intuition and metacognition in medical education.* New York, NY: Spring.

Schmidt, H. G., & Boshuizen, P. A. (1993). On acquiring expertise in medicine. *Educational Psychology Review, 5*(3), 205–221.

Tversky, A., & Khaneman, D. (1974). Judgment under uncertainty: Heuristics and biases. *Science, 185,* 1124–1131.

Wagner, R. K., & Sternberg, R. J. (1985). Practical intelligence in real-world pursuits: The role of tacit knowledge. *Journal of Personality and Psychology, 49*(2), 436–458.

17

Emotional Labor, Compassion Fatigue, Stress, and Burnout

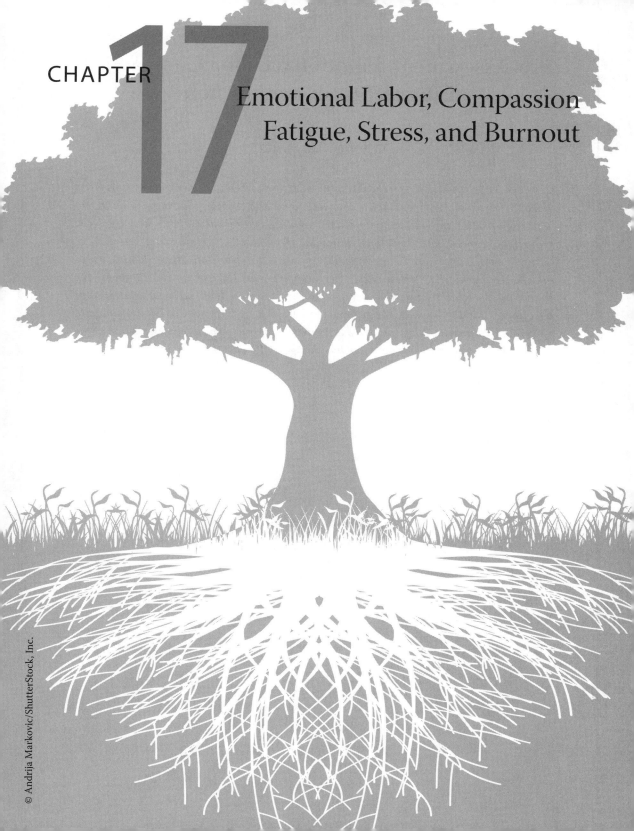

Pre-Assessment: Emotional Labor, Compassion Fatigue, Stress, and Burnout

Mind Mapping

Consider the terms arrayed on the page. For each term, without thinking or editing, write down the ideas, concepts, examples, contradictions, and theories that come to mind. Do not array them in any systematic or orderly manner. Scatter them about the page. Now, draw lines between your additions, indicating that there is a relationship between the terms. If something causes something else, indicate this with an arrow. Relationships may be reciprocal—both cause each other—requiring arrows at both ends. Indicate the strength of the relationship by darkening and thickening the lines; stronger relationships have darker and thicker lines. Most important: There is no right answer. Do not compare with your classmates. *What you have is a mind map, your mental representation of the topic. Review to determine if anything has changed following this section.*

Emotional labor
Compassion fatigue
Stress
Burnout

⧈ DESIRED EDUCATIONAL OUTCOMES

- Discuss the concept of emotional labor and the dissonance associated with it.
- Explain the concept of compassion fatigue.
- Discuss the impact of stress on performance and quality of life.
- Consider the impact of stress on professional obligation.

⧈ DESIRED PERSONAL OUTCOME

- Achieve an enhanced ability to deal with stress.

Emotional Labor

CONSUMERS AND PATIENTS EVALUATE SERVICE encounters based not only on the reliability and timeliness of the service, but also on the emotions displayed by the service provider. Was the waitress friendly, the ticket taker pleasant, or the pharmacist empathic? Do I, as the consumer, feel that the pharmacist cared about me and my circumstances? When I conveyed my situation was the reaction appropriate; was it genuine? For a few moments could I feel that the pharmacist cared about me, or did I sense I was an interruption? Did they smile where appropriate, furl their eyebrows at the right point, and seem saddened by my loss? Service jobs in general, and health care in particular, require practitioners to regulate their emotions to fit the circumstances. The original work in this field, *The Managed Heart* (2003), captured this idea. This emotional requirement is termed *emotional labor*. Emotional labor is when feelings are changed or masked based on specific organizational requirements.

In any situation the healthcare provider's emotional state may be either congruent (felt and expressed emotions are consistent) or discordant (felt and expressed emotions are different). Two emotional labor strategies result in congruent emotional states. Those strategies are:

- *Deep acting:* In deep acting, the individual internalizes the required emotional reaction. Initially the individual may have to modify their felt emotions so that what is presented on the outside matches what is inside. There may be an initial discordance, but with the investment of time and energy this discordance is resolved. Think of someone initially repelled by a class of patients who grows to care for them and displays that concern.

- *Emotional consonance:* The individual's natural emotions are in line with what is expected. Generally, individuals have a natural affinity and compassion for small babies; thus, displaying the appropriate emotional reactions is genuine.

One emotional labor strategy results in a discordant emotional state. That strategy is:

- *Surface acting:* This involves presenting a façade, putting on a mask because what is shown is what is expected. With surface acting true emotions are not modified. Think of having to act polite and concerned while a patient rants and raves at you. With surface acting the emotional dissonance is never resolved. Alternatively, the emotions may simply be suppressed.

In meeting the "feeling rules" for the situation, pharmacists may have to suppress their anxiety, anger, fear, and dislike to display calm, kindness, and empathy. Over time emotional dissonance may become debilitating, leading to both physiological and psychological problems. Emotional labor, particularly when dissonant, may lead to burnout, affect job satisfaction, increase intent to leave, and negatively impact performance. Those who engage in surface acting without ever resolving the tension between felt and required emotions are most likely to experience these negative consequences.

Compassion Fatigue

"COMPASSION FATIGUE DESCRIBES THE EMOTIONAL, physical, social, and spiritual exhaustion that overtakes a person and causes a pervasive decline in his or her desire, ability, and energy to feel and care for others" (McHolm, 2006, p. 12). Compassion fatigue is a result of helping others in distress. As a result, the caregiver is traumatized. Compassion fatigue is similar to burnout. Burnout is progressive and results in indifference, disengagement, and withdrawal. Compassion fatigue is sometimes acute in onset, though the underlying stresses often build over time, and may result in overinvolvement with the patient. Compassion fatigue is often character-ized by a sense of helplessness and confusion. It is the result of high levels of involvement with a patient without the compensating reward of seeing improvement. Pharmacists involved with end-of-life care would be likely candidates for suffering from compassion fatigue. The symptoms of com-passion fatigue are (adapted from Lombardo & Eyre, 2011):

- *Work-related:* Avoidance or dread of working with certain patients, reduced ability to feel empathy towards patients or families, frequent use of sick days, lack of joyfulness

- *Physical:* headaches, digestive problems, muscle tension, sleep dis-turbances, fatigue, cardiac symptoms

- *Emotional:* Mood swings; restlessness; irritability; oversensitivity; anxiety; depression; anger and resentment; loss of objectivity; mem-ory issues; excessive use of alcohol, nicotine, or illicit drugs; poor concentration, focus, or judgment

Though any single symptom may indicate compassion fatigue, generally more than one symptom is required to confirm this assessment.

Burnout

THE DEVELOPMENT OF BURNOUT IS often insidious. It is similar to the frog in the beaker where the temperature gradually rises so that it doesn't realize it is being boiled. Burnout involves the loss of idealism, energy, and purpose. In burnout, mental and physical resources are gradu-ally depleted. Different levels of burnout may develop. First-level burnout is relatively mild, transient, and occasional. Mid-level burnout is more stable, lasts longer, and is more difficult to eradicate. Third-level burnout is charac-terized by symptoms that are chronic and accompanied by a physical illness. All health professionals suffer first-level burnout during the course of a year; most experience mid-level burnout sometimes, and a few move on to level three. Those experiencing burnout often attribute this feeling to a personal deficiency, that *something is wrong with me.*

A key psychological point regarding burnout is to recognize that no matter what goes on around you, you ultimately control your response to it. A feeling of powerlessness is a critical contributor to burnout. Beyond this, the key recommendation for dealing with burnout is balance, primarily the balance in taking care of the patient and taking care of yourself. The same balance extends to your personal life. Your professional obligation demands that you give *of* yourself, but it also demands that you give *to* yourself. Without the appropriate level of giving to yourself, ultimately patient care suffers.

Balance can be summarized as a blend of compassion and objectivity characterized by detached concern. There is an appropriate level of involvement. Being close allows the practitioner to see the patient as a fellow human being rather than a statistic. Being objective allows the practitioner to bring intellectual powers and professional insight to bear, devoid of emotional bias. Being distant allows the practitioner to see the patient as a case. The shrewd clinician maintains the appropriate balance of each, and moves from one to the other as required.

The ultimate question is, who will help the helper? Although help is often available at some level from various sources, the point to remember is that most often you will be your own helper.

Stress and Quality of Life

STRESS IS THE BODY'S REACTION to any demand. In other words, it is a response to something happening in the environment. Stress at work is due to such things as workload, lack of control, and uncertainty as to what is required. Stress is related to job satisfaction, intent to leave, and absenteeism. Workplace stress also has physiological effects such as high blood pressure, fatigue, insomnia, and headaches. In short, workplace stress is a significant contributor to whether or not a job is satisfying. It is not a question of if there will be stress, but when and what toll it will take. The key impediment to dealing with stress is denial. Realizing that self-care is not a waste of time or a sign of weakness is the next step.

Suggestions for self-care and self-comfort follow (adapted from Dahlqvist, Soderberg, & Norberg, 2008):

- *Unload* by getting things off your chest. Have the courage to admit your fears and vulnerabilities, the things that frustrate you and anger you, in a safe, private environment.

- *Distract* yourself with other activities, such as exercising, reading, watching movies, and so on. Don't do so to the point of avoidance, but create a brief space to crystallize feelings, thoughts, and options.

- *Nurture* yourself with a small treat, focusing on your needs.

- *Withdraw* from the fray for a while; disconnect the phone, avoid emails, and be out of contact.

- *Reassure* yourself of your value, worth, and contributions.

- *Find new perspectives* on the circumstance; view the circumstance from a different angle.

Stress and Performance

STRESS ALSO HAS A SIGNIFICANT impact on performance. In one view, stress has a negative impact on performance because time and energy are consumed in dealing with the stress. Also, stress tends to narrow perceptions, resulting in missed information. Concern over the physiological reactions to stress also narrows focus. Another view suggests that stress is beneficial to performance because individuals respond to the increased challenges of the situation. In this view, performance suffers if the individual is not challenged, or stressed. A third view combines both perspectives, resulting in an inverted-U response to stress (Muse, Harris, & Feild, 2003). As stress increases from low levels to some peak, performance increases. Beyond this peak, performance declines as the debilitating aspects of stress emerge.

A clinician's reaction to stress, or lack of a reaction, is an insight with implications for impacting patient outcomes. Some clinicians may find the stress of a high volume pharmacy operation intolerable, whereas others take it in stride. Some clinicians may be energized by the feeling of walking on the edge in an intensive care setting, whereas others will be rendered ineffective by the high stakes and time-constrained demands of this setting. It is unlikely that any practice setting will be devoid of performance-related stress; learning to deal with the peculiar stresses of that setting is a professional obligation.

The lessons from psychology for improving performance include the following (adapted from Hays, 2009):

- *Relaxation:* Many problems relating to performance under stress stem from the anxiety associated with performance. Think of how you would converse with your colleagues in a relaxed setting versus how you would converse with them as a panel discussion in front of 500 colleagues at a professional meeting. The goal is to turn down the impact of the sympathetic nervous system. Relaxation can be learned as well as trained for.

- *Self-talk:* The goal is not to talk yourself out of performing well. Self-talk such as "I will never pass this test," or "No one will accept my recommendations" is self-defeating. Self-talk is used to reframe circumstances and cast them in a positive light.

- *Imagery:* The concept is to picture yourself accomplishing your objective—for example, visualizing yourself passing the NAPLEX.

- *Goal setting and concentration:* Establishing outcome goals is always helpful. Establishing process goals may be even more helpful; for example, staying focused and concentrating on the present, saying what do I have to do now?

The key point is that one can learn to overcome the debilitating performance aspects of stress. Tennis players can learn to swing out on the match points. Similarly, you can learn how to perform under the probing questions of the chief of staff on rounds, or how to take a high stakes exam and do well.

Resilience

RESILIENCE IS THE ABILITY TO respond to both acute and chronic stress in a manner that is effective. Those responses are cognitive, emotional, and behavioral. Resilience is the ability to "keep on keeping on." It is not a quality of the few; rather, its practice is within the grasp of everyone. Attitude is at the heart of resilience. The intent to remain in control, to persevere, to overcome, and to win is the key. The specific strengths that underlie resilience are as follows (adapted from Neenan, 2009):

- *High frustration tolerance* is the ability to endure without lapsing into self-pity, to accept the inherent discomfort. Suffering and discomfort are endured in pursuit of a goal, not for their own sake or to demonstrate your toughness.

- *Self-acceptance* is an understanding that you are both talented and flawed, accomplished and deficient, empathic and insensitive—a complex mixture of attributes. Self-acceptance avoids rating yourself as good or bad. You are just you.

- *Self-belief* is the understanding that you can accomplish what you need to. Self-belief results from having established goals and then doing what is necessary to accomplish those goals.

- *Humor* is the defense against taking yourself and your circumstances too seriously. Seeing the absurdity in much of what we do opens the valve to release the building internal pressure.

- *Problem-solving skills* involve removing the internal and external blocks to getting things done.

- *Finding meaning* is the bridge between the tedium of today and the grand future and promise of tomorrow—a diaper changed is a graduating son or daughter someday.

Stress at Work

THE FOLLOWING IS A SAMPLE scenario related to stress involving RPG (recent pharmacy graduate):

RPG had gone to work for a small group of independent pharmacies in a rural part of the state. The owners of the pharmacy had spent their entire careers building from one store to the current seven stores. RPG had heard about and understood the sacrifices and struggles that had been made to accomplish this. RPG felt a distinct obligation to perform in such a manner so he could help to continue this growth.

RPG had been given the assignment of coordinating the purchase of antibiotics for the upcoming winter season. This involved coordinating the requests from each of the stores and then calculating the best option, taking into account predicted demand, storage space, terms regarding payment, discounts earned, and return policies. RPG worked on this project for over a month after hours at home. The last time RPG felt this way was while working full time and preparing for the NAPLEX. The tension was almost overwhelming. RPG began to feel that if he made mistakes the company might be at risk. RPG knew that margins were continuing to decline. The talk among the owners was always cash flow and profitability, and he overheard they might be forced to let one pharmacist go if trends continued. RPG was the last pharmacist hired, and so he assumed it would be him. He also knew that two of the pharmacies were located in small towns over 30 miles from the nearest pharmacy. Should one of these stores close, RPG understood the hardships that would be imposed on their elderly patients. RPG started to obsess about getting it right. He often woke up in the middle of the night thinking about the situation and found that his weekly golf was less enjoyable. RPG felt guilty about taking the leisure time when he should be working on the project. RPG caught himself almost making mistakes at work as his mind wandered back to the purchasing project.

How would you recommend RPG handle the situation?

Assignment: What Do the Practitioners/ Others Say?

B E PREPARED TO DISCUSS EMOTIONAL labor, compassion fatigue, stress, and burnout based on any *one* of the following:

- A discussion with your colleagues, or others, on how they feel and what they know about emotional labor, compassion fatigue, stress, and burnout

- An article on emotional labor, compassion fatigue, stress, and burnout, either from the research literature or any other source

- A movie/television program/YouTube video about emotional labor, compassion fatigue, stress, and burnout

- A book on emotional labor, compassion fatigue, stress, and burnout (literary, historical, psychological, or any other source)

EXERCISES

1. Discuss with several of your classmates your particular strategies for dealing with test anxiety. Describe what you say to yourself before you take a test. Describe what you say to yourself after you receive the grade.

2. View the original movie *M*A*S*H* and observe how the staff dealt with stress, fatigue, and burnout. Which of their choices were appropriate, and which were not? Discuss your observations with several of your classmates.

⫸ Thick Face/Black Heart: What Do You Think?

The Asian concept of face refers to how others think of you. It is a concern that others think well of you. The western idea of a thick skin is a lack of concern with criticism and what others think of you. Merging both ideas approximates the idea of thick face: "a shield to protect our self-esteem from the bad opinions of others" (Chu, 1992, p. 10). Those with thick face eliminate self-doubt and do not accept external or self-imposed limitations. Thick face is a shield from the debilitating opinions of others.

Having a black heart is ruthlessness in the pursuit of a goal, but not necessarily evil. Successful amputations pre-anesthesia required a surgeon who cut swiftly and decisively without concern for the patient's screams. Success required a callousness to the feelings of another. Black-hearted individuals have the courage to fail. They do what has to be done.

At the crudest level, thick face/black heart has no moral restrictions; it is winning at all costs. This stage is winning, but not victory. With time, the individual recognizes the bankruptcy of this approach and embarks on a period of self-discovery and begins the transition to a phase of dispassion and detachment. In this stage, the individual recognizes life (professional practice) is a battle to be fought. It is the ability to execute our obligations with wisdom based on a personal self-mastery. Conquering ourselves, we can then conquer our circumstances.

Is this relevant to the prior chapters on success, failure, and mistakes and to the discussion in this chapter on stress and performance? If so, how? If not, why?

⊪ Emotional Labor

Please answer the following questions using this scale:
1 = strongly agree; 2 = disagree; 3 = slightly disagree; 4 = slightly agree; 5 = agree; 6 = strongly agree

1. I often pretend to have the emotions I need to show for clients. (SA)

2. I often "put on an act" in order to deal with clients. (SA)

3. I often find myself faking to clients that I am in a good mood. (SA)

4. I can create a look of concern for a client, when in reality I am not concerned. (SA)

5. When dealing with a difficult client I can put on a sympathetic face, even though in reality I am feeling irritated. (SA)

SA = surface acting

Higher scores indicate levels of emotional labor and emotional labor strategies utilized.

Source: Blau, G., Fertig, J., Tatum D. S., Connaughton, S., Park, D. S., & Marshall, C. (2010). Further scale refinement for emotional labor. *Career Development International*, *15*(2), 198.

Based on your responses, write a one-paragraph description of yourself as it relates to emotional labor, compassion fatigue, stress, and burnout.

⊪ Burnout and Stress and the Emotional Intelligence Framework

Have you ever worked in a pharmacy during the height of the flu season? What happens to performance and service after 2–3 weeks of overload work? If you have never experienced this, consider what the semester would be like if the stress of finals lasted for 15 weeks.

Self-aware: Describe your reaction to stress at work. Describe your reaction to stress in your personal life. Consider the impact of stress on your body, and on your mental state.

Self-management: In the past, how have you handled stress? What improvements could you make in how you deal with stress?

Social awareness: Observe one or two people at work or in your personal life and how they manage stress. What can you learn from their approach?

Relationship management: How are your relationships altered when you are stressed? If you are stressed, does being tired, hungry, or drinking have an impact on your relationships?

⑾ **Personal Learning Plan: Burnout and Stress**

These steps can be compiled on a single page containing the following:

What prompted me to develop this plan?

What is the general area for improvement?

What is the specific issue for improvement?

Why is this important to me?

How do I generally act in these areas?

What are my goals?

What prompted this effort?

What strategies are required?

Who/what is necessary to meet my goals with this strategy?

How will I measure the success/failure of this effort?

How long will I focus on this effort?

How will I reflect and capture a lesson from this effort that can be generalized to other circumstances.

✦ WHAT'S IMPORTANT TO YOU IN THE CHAPTER?

With several of your classmates, discuss the idea/ideas that are most likely to effect change in your values, attitudes, or behaviors. Be succinct—no more than two sentences.

✦ REFERENCES

Blau, G., Fertig, J., Tatum D. S., Connaughton, S., Park, D. S., & Marshall, C. (2010). Further scale refinement for emotional labor. *Career Development International*, *15*(2), 188–216.

Chu, C.-N., (1992). *Thick face—Black heart*. New York, NY: Warner.

Dahlqvist, V., Soderberg, A., & Norberg, A. (2008). Dealing with stress: Patterns of self-comfort among healthcare students. *Nurse Education Today*, *28*, 476–484.

Hays, K. F. (2009). *Performance psychology in action*. Washington, DC: American Psychological Association.

Lombardo, B., & Eyre, C. (2011). Compassion fatigue: A nurse's primer. *Online Journal of Issues in Nursing*, *16*(1). http://www.nursingworld.org/MainMenuCategories/ANAMarketplace /ANAPeriodicals/OJIN TableofContents/Vol-16-2011/No1-Jan-2011 /Compassion-Fatigue-A-Nurses-Primer.html.

McHolm, F. (2006). Rx for compassion fatigue. *Journal of Christian Nursing*, *23*(4), 12–19.

Muse, L. A., Harris, S. G., & Feild, H. S. (2003). Has the inverted-U theory of stress and job performance had a fair test? *Human Performance*, *16*(4), 349–364.

Neenan, M. (2009). *Developing resilience*. London, UK: Routledge.

✦ SUGGESTED READINGS

Figley, C. R. (2002). *Treating compassion fatigue*. New York, NY: Brunner-Routledge.

Hochschild, A. R. (2003). *The managed heart: The commercialization of feeling*. London, England: University of California Press.

251

Holmes, E. (2008, March). *The role of emotional dissonance as an affective state on the emotional labor process of retail chain pharmacists* (Unpublished doctoral dissertation). Oxford, MS: University of Mississippi.

Karim, J., & Weisz, R. (2011). Emotional intelligence as a moderator of affectivity/emotional labor and emotional labor/psychological stress. *Psychological Studies, 56*(4), 348–359.

Lapane, K. L., & Hughes, C. M. (2004). Baseline job satisfaction and stress among pharmacists and pharmacy technicians participating in the Fleetwood Phase III study. *Consultant Pharmacist, 19*(11), 1029–1037.

Lea, V. M., Corlett, S. A., & Rodgers, R. M. (2012). Workload and its impact on community pharmacists' job satisfaction and stress; a review of the literature. *International Journal of Pharmacy Practice, 20*(4), 259–271.

Mann, S. (2005). A health-care model of emotional labour: An evaluation of the literature and development of a model. *Journal of Health Organization and Management, 19*(4/5), 304–317.

Maslach, C. (1982). *Burnout—The cost of caring.* Englewood Cliffs, NJ: Prentice Hall.

Mesmer-Magnus, J. R., DeChurch, L. A., & Wax, A. (2011). Moving emotional labor beyond surface and deep acting: A discordance-congruence perspective. *Organizational Psychology Review, 2*(1), 6–53.

Mockler, R. J., & Dologite, D. G. (1999). Learning how to learn: Nurturing professional growth through cognitive mapping. *New England Journal of Entrepreneurship, 2*(2), 65–80.

Reid, L. D., Motycka, C., Mobley, C., & Meldrum, M. (2006). Comparing self-reported burnout of pharmacy students on the founding campus with those at a distance campus. *American Journal of Pharmacy Education, 70*(5), 1–12.

Rothschild, B. (2006). *Help for the helper.* New York, NY: Norton.

Stamm, B. H. (2009). Professional quality of life: Compassion satisfaction and fatigue (ProQOL) Version 5. Retrieved from http://www.proqol.org/uploads/ProQOL_5_English.pdf.

Wharton, A. S. (2009). The sociology of emotional labor. *Annual Review of Sociology, 35*, 147–165.

Wicks, R. J. (2006). *Overcoming secondary stress in medical and nursing practice.* Oxford, UK: Oxford University Press.

Wicks, R. J. (2008). *The resilient clinician.* Oxford, UK: Oxford University Press.

CHAPTER 18

Establishing Credibility

Pre-Assessment: Establishing Credibility

Mind Mapping

Consider the terms arrayed on the page. For each term, without thinking or editing, write down the ideas, concepts, examples, contradictions, and theories that come to mind. Do not array them in any systematic or orderly manner. Scatter them about the page. Now, draw lines between your additions, indicating that there is a relationship between the terms. If something causes something else, indicate this with an arrow. Relationships may be reciprocal—both cause each other—requiring arrows at both ends. Indicate the strength of the relationship by darkening and thickening the lines; stronger relationships have darker and thicker lines. Most important: There is no right answer. Do not compare with your classmates. *What you have is a mind map, your mental representation of the topic. Review to determine if anything has changed following this section.*

Establishing credibility
Entitlement
First impressions
Personal presence

⦚ DESIRED EDUCATIONAL OUTCOMES

- Discuss the impact of openness to experience on establishing credibility.
- Discuss establishing credibility at work.
- Explain self-efficacy and credibility.
- Consider establishing a presence at work.

⦚ DESIRED PERSONAL OUTCOME

- Enhance personal credibility at work.

The Objective

IN THE BUSINESS WORLD, THE BCG Growth-Share Matrix is famous. The matrix allows a strategist to classify business units based on their relative market share and market growth rate. The same type of matrix can be adapted to categorize practitioners. This revised matrix substitutes potential professional growth for market growth rate and current skill level for relative market share (see **Figure 18.1**). (Note: The terminology used to describe practitioners in the following text is that of the BCG matrix. It is not meant to demean individuals.) Practitioners with a high potential for growth and high current skill levels would be stars. Time and assets will be required to develop their high potential, but the end result will be a top-flight practitioner. Those with high skill levels but a low potential for growth would be workhorses. These practitioners have maximized their capabilities and are valuable contributors. Those with low potential for growth and low current skill levels would be dogs; these are practitioners that are a drain on operations. Those with a high potential for growth but low current skill levels are question marks—it is not clear whether they will ever develop into an effective practitioner. Establishing credibility is about being recognized for your personal, professional, and clinical competence; or your potential in these areas. The objective for a new practitioner should be to be recognized as either a star or a question mark.

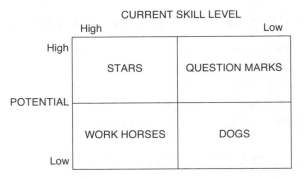

Figure 18.1

Establishing Credibility

A S A NEW PRACTITIONER, NO one should expect you to perform as if you have been practicing for 10 years. Trying to convey that you can function at this level is a mistake. Displaying certain attitudes and behaviors will establish your credibility. The first is curiosity and a willingness to learn all that is required to be effective as a clinician, as an employee, and as a colleague. Although no one should expect you to know everything, they will expect you to be enthused about your current circumstances. No task should be beneath you. In fact, you may be assigned some undesirable tasks as a test. Accept the requests graciously and do your best. Insisting that being a Doctor of Pharmacy insulates you from some of the dirty work will poison relationships. Think of these tasks as a rite of passage. Related to this point, be cautious about insisting on being addressed by your formal title. In certain circumstances, a more formal protocol is warranted; however, in private, respectful familiarity is appropriate. The second aspect of establishing credibility is to convey that you can be trusted. In this arena, actions speak louder than words. Doing what you say you will and on time is the standard. Finally, credibility is about being liked. Generally, people like to work with people who are similar to them, they are familiar with, have reciprocal positive feelings, and are attractive, either in appearance or personality. People like working with people who are cheerful, considerate, and generous. Research has shown that if someone is strongly disliked, whether they are competent or not is irrelevant; no one will work with them. In contrast, if someone is liked, coworkers will seek out every aspect of their competence (Casciaro & Lobo, 2005). In other words, being liked earns you the benefit of the doubt as to competence.

Successful opening days of a career require managing the initial impression you present. Strategies for managing impressions include (adapted from Turnley & Bolino, 2001):

- *Ingratiation:* Praising others for their efforts, complimenting others, doing favors, taking an interest in others' personal lives
- *Self-promotion:* Letting others know of your talents and qualifications, how valuable you are, and relating past accomplishments
- *Exemplification:* Letting others know how hard you work, taking on more than your share of work, arriving early and staying late
- *Supplication:* Trying to gain sympathy so others will help you, acting like you know less than you do to get help, disclosing your weaknesses
- *Intimidation:* Letting others know you won't be pushed around, dealing forcefully with others to do things your way

Using supplication and intimidation are not recommended because one is likely to appear either needy and lazy or bossy. Handled correctly, ingratiation leads others to see you as likeable, self-promotion leads others to see you as competent, and exemplification leads others to see you as dedicated. Handled poorly, ingratiation leads others to see you as a sycophant, self-promotion leads others to see you as conceited, and exemplification leads others to see you as feeling superior.

Personal insecurity and institutional pressures to perform may entice new practitioners to behave in the way they are "supposed to" in professional situations. Such felt obligations to behave in specified ways may lead the new practitioners to try to impress others in ways that are not appropriate; the negatives of impression management detailed previously result. Describing research you were involved with as a student establishes your credibility in an area; boasting of its significance likely hides your insecurity. Behaving authentically is the shield from making these mistakes. You need to be self-aware enough to know what you are feeling and what your values are, and astute enough to frame your behaviors and your sent impressions based on this—based on being authentic. Behavior at work is assuming a role; in some aspects it is playing a part. The art is to not overact. If it feels fake to you—it is.

Openness to Experience

N O MATTER HOW MANY HOURS a student has accumulated working as a pharmacy technician or as an intern, the first day as a licensed practitioner is different; it will feel different. The staff will be looking to you for decisions, for direction. What is the objective in the very first stages of a new career? It is to establish credibility, to earn the trust of those you will be working for, with, and directing. The task is to minimize any missteps in the first few days of practice that might taint perceptions of your competence. This task will be shaped by the individual's relative openness to experience. For those relatively high on the personality dimension of openness to experience, this task will be easier; for others, it will be more of a challenge. Those more open to experience tend to be more receptive to change and are more willing to try new things, as well as tolerate divergent views. They are inquisitive and open to feedback about themselves. Those high in this personality dimension are more likely to adopt a learning goal orientation and develop effective learning strategies. Displaying enthusiasm and receptivity to learning how things are done in a new job, to being open, is the first step in establishing credibility.

Perceived Self-Efficacy

S ELF-EFFICACY IS THE BELIEF THAT one can cope with adversity and accomplish difficult or novel tasks. It is the belief that you can do the job. If you do not believe you are capable of developing into a competent professional and clinician, then it is unlikely you ever will. Personal self-efficacy is a self-appraisal of one's capabilities. Personal self-efficacy derives from four sources:

1. Having been successful in other aspects of your life; in short, success enhances self-efficacy.

2. Vicarious experience; if they can do it, then so can I.

3. Encouragement from others about your ability. Having someone say, "You can do it!"

4. Emotional and physiological factors; if I am nervous with butterflies in my stomach before meeting a stranger, then I must not be good at it.

Individuals have a generalized sense of self-efficacy about themselves—their global assessment of themselves and specific self-efficacy assessments. It is the belief that in general you are competent, but not adept at certain tasks. For others to believe you are competent, you must first believe it about yourself.

First Impressions

WE HAVE COMPLETE CONTROL OVER how we present ourselves—how we dress, our facial expressions, our posture and physical presence, our hairstyles, and the like. What we don't control is the perceptions others have of us. Others view us through filters, lens, and influences that may distort their perceptions. Those filters include meta programs—the way people think and their approach to thinking. A meta program is the way a person handles information. Some people value substance over style, some are deep thinkers, others respond to surface attributes. Some people are engineers and others are artists. A second filter is a person's belief system—their view or theory of the world. A third filter is a person's values—their definition of what is right or wrong, good or bad. The fourth filter is a person's memories—the things they have lived through and experienced. The final filter is the person's past decisions. Decisions made in the past and whether they worked or not continue to color a person's world into the future. One colleague may find your very expensive and stylish clothes a waste of money whereas another sees them as a marker of someone interested in the newest and latest, and views that as an indicator of progressivism. Professional colleagues in mid-town New York, Chicago, and Boston will most likely view you with different filters than professional colleagues in rural South Dakota or Montana. Calculate and calibrate your first impression with an eye toward the audience. There is never an opportunity to make another first impression.

Personal Presence

I N HER BOOK, *CREATING PERSONAL PRESENCE*, Dianna Booher asked how much personal presence affects credibility. The response from 74.5 percent of the respondents was, a great deal. Developing presence is no mystery. It is based on the following:

- *How you look:* Body language, handshake, movement, dress, energy, personal space

- *How you talk:* The words you choose, how you use your voice, the ability to carry on a conversation, emotional outbursts and reactions

- *How you think:* How you organize your ideas, what you say, what you withhold, how you frame problems, your ability to think on your feet under pressure, your ability to communicate with stories

- *How you act:* The attitudes, values, and competence your actions convey; being genuine; acting with integrity; being thoughtful; having a sense of humor; being competent and accountable

How you look and talk are the most observable and least important aspects. How you think and act are the least observable but most important. When you graduate you will have a choice in these matters. You can opt to express your freedom from external expectations and constraints. Or, you can opt to express your professionalism, your maturity, and your understanding that for the patient and your colleagues the superficial and the obvious are all that they have to judge you on. Your character is the basis for your personal presence, but it is impossible for others to perceive what is in your heart.

Although what is in your heart cannot be assessed, your cyber-footprint can be. Given the ubiquitous nature of the Internet and social media, caution as to what is uploaded is in order. Although you might believe that your postings are private and intended for personal audiences and acquaintances only, this may not be the case. Further, your postings are eternal. When applying for a director of pharmacy job in 20 years, will the comments you make today reflect a consummate professional or a relatively immature college student whose judgment is clouded by alcohol or youthful indiscretion? Your personal presence and credibility are functions of how you look, talk, think, and act. They are also functions of what you post.

A Sense of Entitlement

ALL PEOPLE ARE A PRODUCT of their specific culture and place in history. For some, your great-grandparents were shaped by the Depression and World War II; for others, your grandparents were influenced by the conformity of the 1950s and the turbulence of the 1960s. Many students today have been shaped by the following forces: mothers who worked outside the home, parents who waited later to have children, spending time in daycare and with babysitters, the use of television and the Internet for entertainment and as a substitute for family interaction, parents who hovered about and protected them and often lavished unwarranted praise. Many positive attributes are associated with today's students: goal oriented, socially conscious, technologically proficient. However, certain negative traits also are associated with today's students: self-absorbed, overprotected, low frustration tolerance, requiring focused and immediate feedback, seeking constant feedback, and entitled. As a new practitioner, an awareness of these traits is important. The people you will be working for most likely will view the world from the perspective of a different generation. Entitlement is an expectation of success without a personal responsibility for achieving that success. Entitlement may be a natural feeling for today's student, but expressing that sense of entitlement during the first few days of work is a recipe for stepping off on the wrong foot.

Credibility at Work

THE FOLLOWING ARE SAMPLE SCENARIOS related to credibility involving RPG (recent pharmacy graduate):

RPG was asked to interview two potential students for the hospital's residency program. She reviewed the two files in front of her. The first interviewee walked into the office and introduced herself. She was attractive and professionally dressed in a business suit. She smiled, her demeanor was pleasant and engaged, and she exuded a sense of compassion and empathy. She asked about RPG's class ring and what school had been like for her. She answered questions directly, and was candid enough to answer "I don't know" to one question and asked for a moment or two for consideration before answering another question. She indicated she really wanted the residency and was prepared to leave her fiancé in another city for a year to take the position. Her grades were good but not outstanding. RPG felt an immediate connection with this applicant.

The second interviewee came highly recommended from a former professor, and her grades were outstanding. The second interviewee walked in and said that she felt like you already knew each other because she had talked to RPG's mutual former professor about her. She neglected to introduce herself or shake hands. She was dressed in a business suit that was expensive but not well tailored. The interviewee asked to be called by her nickname. When asked a question she couldn't answer, she seemed to lose her poise. Her responses seemed calculated and guarded. She seemed mostly concerned about the expectations for the residency. She indicated what a big sacrifice it would be to move away from her family to accept the residency. Although RPG and this candidate had gone to the same school and her answers were right, they didn't feel genuine.

How would you recommend RPG handle the situation?

During the first week of work, RPG made a recommendation that in the moment seemed right and appeared to be taken under advisement and accepted by the attending physician. That evening, RPG continued going over the case in his mind and realized that although his recommendation was not incorrect, there was a preferred course of action.

How would you recommend RPG handle the situation?

Assignment: What Do the Practitioners/Others Say?

BE PREPARED TO DISCUSS ESTABLISHING credibility based on any *one* of the following:

- A discussion with your colleagues, or others, on how they feel and what they know about establishing credibility

- An article on establishing credibility, from either the research literature or any other source

- A movie/television program/YouTube video about establishing credibility

- A book on establishing credibility (literary, historical, psychological, or any other source)

EXERCISES

◀▌▶ What If You Don't Know?

With several of your classmates, discuss the best way to handle the situation when you don't know the answer. What if the questioner is a doctor? A nurse? A patient?

◀▌▶ First Impressions

With several of your classmates, discuss the best way to make a first impression. What advice would you give?

◀▌▶ Personal Presence

Ask yourself how you would assess your competence and professionalism based on your personal presence—how you look, talk, think, and act. Ask your classmates, family, and friends to do the same thing.

◀▌▶ Externalized Responsibility Subscale

Please answer the questions using the following scale:
1 = strongly disagree; 2 = disagree; 3 = somewhat disagree; 4 = neither agree or disagree; 5 = somewhat agree; 6 = agree; 7 = strongly agree

1. It is unnecessary for me to participate in class when the professor is paid for teaching, not for asking questions. _____

2. If I miss class, it is my responsibility to get the notes. *(Reverse)* _____

3. I am not motivated to put a lot of effort into group work, because another group member will end up doing it. _____

4. I believe that the university does not provide me with the resources I need to succeed in college. _____

5. Most professors do not really know what they are talking about. _____

6. If I do poorly in a course and I could not make my professor's office hours, the fault lies with my professor. _____

7. I believe that it is my responsibility to seek out the resources to succeed in college. *(Reverse)* _____

8. For group assignments, it is acceptable to take a back seat and let others do most of the work if I am busy. _____

9. For group work, I should receive the same grade as the other group members regardless of my level of effort. _____

10. Professors are just employees who get money for teaching. _____

Higher scores indicate a tendency to assign responsibility for outcomes to sources outside yourself. Reverse score: score 7 as 1 or 2 as 6, etc.

Source: Chowning, K., & Campbell, N. J. (2009). Development and validation of a measure of academic entitlement: Individual differences in students' externalized responsibility and entitled expectations. *Journal of Education Psychology*, *101*(4), 985.

◈ Entitled Expectations Subscale

1. My professors are obligated to help me prepare for exams. _____

2. Professors must be entertaining to be good. _____

3. My professors should reconsider my grade if I am close to the grade I want. _____

4. I should never receive zero on an assignment that I turned in. _____

5. My professors should curve my grade if I am close to the next letter grade. _____

Higher scores indicate a greater sense of academic entitlement.

Source: Chowning, K., & Campbell, N. J. (2009). Development and validation of a measure of academic entitlement: Individual differences in students' externalized responsibility and entitled expectations. *Journal of Education Psychology*, *101*(4), 985.

◈ A Higher Grade

1. In one of your classes you are within a 0.5 percent of a higher grade. What is an entitled response to this situation? What is a personal responsibility response to this situation?

2. In one of your classes you are within 1.0 percent of passing the course. What is an entitled response to this situation? What is a personal responsibility response to this situation?

Based on your responses, write a one-paragraph description of yourself as it relates to establishing credibility.

⫸ Credibility and the Emotional Intelligence Framework

Think of your first job. What was key to establishing credibility in that circumstance?

Self-aware: On a scale from 1 to 10, rate yourself on credibility, and then again on likability. Ask family and friends to rate you.

Self-management: Pick a single personal trait that you could work on to enhance your credibility.

Social awareness: What do you look for in others to determine if you can trust them? To determine if they are credible?

Relationship management: How would you deal with a colleague who you did not believe was credible? How would you deal with a colleague you didn't like? Are these approaches successful?

⫸ Personal Learning Plan: Credibility

These steps can be compiled on a single page containing the following:

What prompted me to develop this plan?

What is the general area for improvement?

What is the specific issue for improvement?

Why is this important to me?

How do I generally act in these areas?

What are my goals?

What prompted this effort?

What strategies are required?

Who/what is necessary to meet my goals with this strategy?

How will I measure the success/failure of this effort?

How long will I focus on this effort?

How will I reflect and capture a lesson from this effort that can be generalized to other circumstances.

✦ WHAT'S IMPORTANT TO YOU IN THE CHAPTER?

With several of your classmates, discuss the idea/ideas that are most likely to effect change in your values, attitudes, or behaviors. Be succinct—no more than two sentences.

✦ REFERENCES

Booher, D. (2011). *Creating personal presence*. San Francisco, CA: Berret-Koehler.

Casciaro, T., & Lobo, S. (2005, June). Competent jerks, lovable fools and the formation of social networks. *Harvard Business Review*, 92–99.

Chowning, K., & Campbell, N. J. (2009). Development and validation of a measure of academic entitlement: Individual differences in students' externalized responsibility and entitled expectations. *Journal of Education Psychology*, *101*(4), 982–997.

Turnley, W. H., & Bolino, M. C. (2001). Achieving desired images while avoiding undesired images: Exploring the role of self-monitoring in impression management. *Journal of Applied Psychology*, *86*(2), 351–360.

✦ SUGGESTED READINGS

Bandura, A. (1993). Perceived self-efficacy in cognitive development and functioning. *Educational Psychologist*, *28*(2), 117–148.

Cain, J., Scott, D. R., & Akers, P. (2009). Pharmacy students' Facebook activity and opinions regarding accountability and e-professionalism. *American Journal of Pharmaceutical Education*, *73*(6), 1–6.

Casciaro, T., & Lobo, M. S. (2008). When competence is irrelevant: The role of interpersonal affect on task-related ties. *Administrative Science Quarterly, 53,* 655–684.

Gjerde, P. F., & Cardilla, K. (2009). Developmental implications of openness to experience in preschool children: Gender differences in young adulthood. *Developmental Psychology, 45*(5), 1455–1464.

Janda, L. (1999). *Career tests.* Avon, MA: Adams Media.

Kelly, P. J. (2010). Age of entitlement; How does physician assistant education change to accommodate the generation Y student? *Journal of Physician Assistant Education, 21*(4), 47–51.

King, G., Currie, M., Baratlett, D. J., Strachan, D., Tucker, M. A., & Willoughby, C. (2008). The development of expertise in paediatric rehabilitation therapists: The roles of motivation, openness to experience, and types of caseload experience. *Australian Occupational Therapy Journal, 55,* 108–122.

Le Pine, J. A., Colquitt, J. A., & Erez, A. (2000). Adaptability to changing task contexts: Effects of general cognitive ability, conscientiousness, and openness to experience. *Personnel Psychology, 53,* 563–593.

Lovas, M., & Holloway, P. (2009). *Axis of influence.* Garden City, NY: Morgan James.

Mavis, B. (2001). Self-efficacy and OSCE performance among second year medical students. *Advances in Health Sciences Education, 6,* 93–102.

Mockler, R. J., & Dologite, D. G. (1999). Learning how to learn: Nurturing professional growth through cognitive mapping. *New England Journal of Entrepreneurship, 2*(2), 65–80.

Wood, A. M., Linley, P. A., Maltby, J., Baliousis, M., & Joseph, S. (2008). The authentic personality test: A theoretical and empirical conceptualization and the development of the authentic scale. *Journal of Counseling Psychology, 55*(3), 385–399.

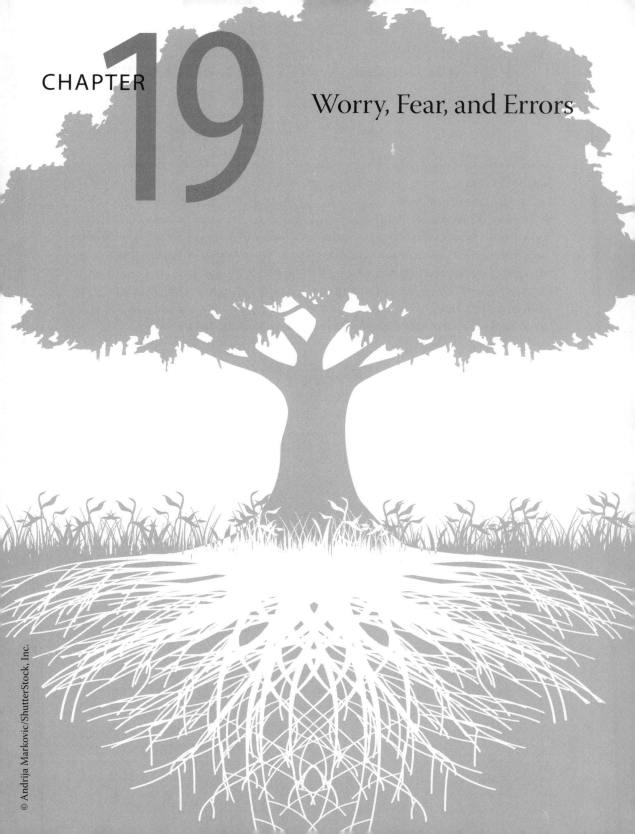

CHAPTER

19

Worry, Fear, and Errors

Pre-Assessment: Worry, Fear, and Errors

Mind Mapping

Consider the terms arrayed on the page. For each term, without thinking or editing, write down the ideas, concepts, examples, contradictions, and theories that come to mind. Do not array them in any systematic or orderly manner. Scatter them about the page. Now, draw lines between your additions, indicating that there is a relationship between the terms. If something causes something else, indicate this with an arrow. Relationships may be reciprocal—both cause each other—requiring arrows at both ends. Indicate the strength of the relationship by darkening and thickening the lines; stronger relationships have darker and thicker lines. Most important: There is no right answer. Do not compare with your classmates. *What you have is a mind map, your mental representation of the topic. Review to determine if anything has changed following this section.*

Worry
Fear of success
Fear of failure
Errors

◆ DESIRED EDUCATIONAL OUTCOMES

- Describe the nature of fear and anxiety.
- Describe the nature of worry.
- Discuss the fear of failure and the fear of success.
- Discuss coping with errors.

◆ DESIRED PERSONAL OUTCOME

- Achieve greater facility and comfort in dealing with the stresses of practice.

Introduction

REMEMBER WHEN YOU MOVED FROM grade school to high school, from high school to college, from the preprofessional phase of pharmacy to the professional sequence? Remember the things you worried about, the things you were afraid of? Soon, the next big transition in your life will take place when you move from a student to a practicing clinician with the attendant responsibilities and obligations. Often accompanying this professional transition are significant changes in your personal life, such as new relationships, moving away from home, buying a house, and so on. It would be the rare individual that doesn't worry about the upcoming changes and soon-to-increase professional and personal responsibilities. This chapter discusses the nature of worry, fear, and anxiety as they relate to clinical practice, with special attention paid to the fear of failure and the fear of medication errors.

Fear and Anxiety

PEOPLE ARE AFRAID OF A lot of things, including ghosts, cockroaches, spiders, snakes, heights, water, enclosed spaces, tunnels, bridges, social rejection, examinations, public speaking, and death. Fear and anxiety are normal reactions to potentially threatening events, either real or imagined. Individuals tend to process the world in a manner consistent with their beliefs about their place in the world and how the world operates. Individuals who are anxious and fearful selectively focus on events that are likely to be harmful; even if the events are nonthreatening or neutral, these people will interpret them as being dangerous. Just as a small child in their room believes there are monsters in the closet or under the bed and scans the ceiling for threatening shadows, excessively anxious and fearful individuals replicate this pattern in their daily lives. Fear is a basic emotion that is universal across all cultures and is hardwired into our DNA (Ekman & Cordaro, 2011). The tendency to excessive fear and anxiety tends to run in families and suggests a genetic component to this pattern. Excessive fear and anxiety are debilitating. An interesting finding is that, "Substantial evidence points to a preponderance of women demonstrating greater fear and anxiety than men across the life span" (McLean & Anderson, 2009, p. 502).

What Is Worry?

WORRY IS THE COGNITIVE COMPONENT of anxiety; it is the anxious apprehension of events. Normal amounts of worry are beneficial. Worry is a legitimate effort to deal with and prepare for potentially stressful events. Worrying about having to make a presentation during rounds is appropriate. Normal worriers attempt to refocus away from the things causing the worry. They attempt to reframe their circumstances in such a way as to minimize their worry. In preparing to make a presentation, a normal worrier might attempt to refocus their attention on some other aspect of their life once their preparations are finalized. Or, a normal worrier might engage in self-talk with a positive theme of, "I will do my best, that is all I can do and they will understand that this is my first presentation, and that I will improve with feedback." Normal and pathological worriers tend to worry about the same types of things. Pathological worriers, however, worry about a greater number of topics, spend more time worrying, and are more likely to worry about minor things. Pathological worriers tend to focus on and look for things to worry about. Pathological worriers will see the "dark side" in any circumstance. Chronic, excessive, uncontrollable worry is central to a diagnosis of generalized anxiety disorder and is often prevalent in depression. Pathological worry is debilitating.

Fear of Failure, Fear of Success

EAR, ANXIETY, AND WORRY CAN be related to innumerable objects, events, individuals, or circumstances. Of particular interest to a new clinician are a fear of failure and the fear and anxiety associated with making an error, particularly one that hurts a patient. Having never been tested in the profession, a fear of failure is appropriate, and the simple statistics suggest that all clinicians/practitioners will ultimately confront the emotional turmoil associated with an error and the aftermath.

Fear of Failure

That people fear failure is intuitively obvious because failure is often accompanied by negative consequences—businesses are lost, courses and tests not passed, spouses leave, promotions are denied, employment is terminated, and so on. The emotional consequences of failure are shame, guilt, and depression. Public humiliation often accompanies failure, and financial losses are often incurred. Hopes and dreams are short circuited, delayed, and denied. Certain fears accompany failure. Generalized fears about failure can be collapsed into the following factors: fear of experiencing shame and embarrassment, fear of devaluing one's self-estimate, fear of having an uncertain future, fear of important others losing interest, and fear of upsetting important others (Conroy, 2001). Fear of failure explains why individuals self-sabotage their efforts by procrastinating or working at less than capacity. This is done to establish an excuse even if they don't do well. Fear of failure also explains why individuals establish goals that are too low when compared with their potential or denigrate their accomplishments when they do succeed. Individuals high in fear of failure may exhibit behavioral patterns characterized as domineering/vindictive or nonassertive/exploitable. Fear of failure is learned, typically in a family situation that is harsh and demanding where love is conditioned on performance. Fear of failure is linked to an excessive or neurotic drive for perfectionism. The mature response to a fear of failure is hard work. In this sense, fear of failure is beneficial.

Fear of Success

It may be counterintuitive, but many people also fear success. Fear of success is a neurotic anxiety about the negative effects of success. For the individual, success may result in social and emotional isolation, guilt over asserting oneself, a fear of discovering true potential, anxiety about surpassing an admired mentor, and a pressure to constantly match or exceed the current performance. As with the fear of failure, those fearing success will self-sabotage or self-handicap themselves to establish psychological defenses if success is not achieved. Women, in particular, may fear success to avoid the psychological tension associated with violating cultural norms and expectations. Also for women, academic success may impact their chances for a successful personal relationship (Coontz, 2012).

Responses to success and failure range from a success orientation to failure acceptance. The specific stages are (adapted from Martin & Marsh, 2003):

- *Success orientation:* Cognitively engaged and behaviorally engaged with success
- *Failure avoidance I (overstriving):* Beginning to engage cognitively with fear of failure but behaviorally engaged with success
- *Failure avoidance II (defensive pessimism):* Cognitively engaged with fear of failure and behaviorally engaged with fear of failure
- *Failure avoidance II (self-handicapping):* Cognitively engaged with fear of failure and behaviorally engaged with fear of failure
- *Failure acceptance (learned helplessness):* Cognitively disengaged and behaviorally disengaged from fear of failure and success

Those engaged with success are optimistic, have a belief and confidence in their ability, believe they are in control, have a focus on learning from mistakes, and are resilient in the face of setbacks. Those seeking to avoid failure are uncertain about their abilities to avoid failure and achieve success, do not believe they are in control, are not resilient in the face of setbacks, and may sabotage their chance for success. Those who accept failure have simply given up, lacking both motivation and resilience.

Errors

"HUMAN ERROR RATES CAN BE reduced to as low a level as desired, at some unknown cost. The occurrence of a particular error at some particular instant, however, cannot absolutely be prevented" (Sender & Moray, 1991, p. 128). In the hospital, patients are probably subjected to one error a day. Most of these are not harmful. However, at least 1.5 million preventable adverse drug events occur each year in the United States. A hospital patient may be subject to one medication error per day (Preventing Medication Errors: Quality Chasm Series, 2007). In 1993, medication errors accounted for 7,000 deaths (Kohn, Corrigan, and Donaldson, 2000). In 2009, 3.9 billion prescriptions were filled in the United States (Kaiser Family Foundation, 2010). Even at an error rate of 1 in 1 million, that means 3,900 errors occur annually. These statistics are for the tangible activity of prescribing, dispensing, and administering medication. Errors in judgment are harder to quantify, as are errors in dealing with patients. Now consider that a community pharmacist could be involved with 200 transactions per day, for 250 days per year, over a 40-year career, or approximately 2 million transactions in a career. The point is that it is highly unlikely any pharmacist will escape their career without being involved in medication errors, some potentially significant or fatal. The focus of this section is on the emotional consequences of those errors and the professional obligations attached to those errors.

Reactions to Errors

Think of your worst performance on an examination, report, or presentation while in pharmacy school. Think of a particularly embarrassing moment from your life, something you shouldn't have said, an inappropriate act, or the like. Now, marry the feelings associated with both. Also, think of having to stand in front of your classmates, friends, and family and let them review your performance in both instances. Finally, the local school paper as well as the informal student grapevine will be abuzz with comments on what happened, how you handled the circumstances, and what it means for your graduation. The point is to have you consider what the likely emotional reaction is to a medication error.

One physician likened the emotional impact of a medical error to entering "the heart of darkness" (Christensen, Levinson, & Dunn, 1992). Errors create a cognitive dissonance for the individual between their self-image as a well-trained, competent professional whose primary goal is to improve patient's lives and someone who has harmed a patient. Errors evoke a wide array of emotional responses that include distress, panic, fear, anger, guilt, shame, humiliation, shock, embarrassment, frustration, grief, excitability, anxiety, and depression. Often these emotional reactions bleed into the practitioner's personal life. These feelings may persist for months and years. Some feelings may never completely disappear because there may be a felt need to continue to punish oneself for the transgression. Self-doubt and loss of confidence are a common psychological residue of an error. At work, relationships with colleagues may be altered. Irritability and curtness in relating to colleagues may occur. Professional reputations are tarnished. Hypervigilence, loss of confidence, and second guessing in performing work-related tasks are likely. Changes in appetite, sleep patterns, and concentration are possible. The intensity of these reactions is generally correlated with the severity of the error. Finally, there is some evidence that for significant errors, women report more stress than men (Waterman et al., 2007, p. 471). A medication error is a life-altering event with the potential to permanently scar the individual.

In one view, those who make errors are considered a "second victim" (Wu et al., 1993). As indicated previously, there is no question that a medication error has a psychological and physical impact on the healthcare provider. The experience of the error and the aftermath tend to follow a predictable trajectory, which is characterized by the stages shown in **Table 19.1**.

Disclosure

THE PATIENT'S DESIRE FOR DISCLOSURE following an error is almost universal. Healthcare providers are motivated to disclose an error to the patient, to self, to the profession, and to the community. Ethics demands that the patient be informed of their health status as a result of an error. The impediment to disclosure is the impact of disclosure on the healthcare provider. Factors that impede disclosing errors include attitudinal barriers such as perfectionism, denial, and arrogance; fears and anxieties such as legal and financial concerns, family reaction, negative publicity, and threat to personal

TABLE 19.1   Error Trajectory

Stage	Stage Characteristics	Common Questions
1: Chaos and response	Error realized. Tell someone. Get help. Deal with patient. Distracted.	How did this happen? Why did this happen?
2: Intrusive response	Reevaluate scenario. Self-isolate. Haunted reenactments. Feelings of inadequacy.	What did I miss? Could it have been prevented?
3: Restoring personal integrity	Managing gossip/grapevine. Fear is prevalent.	What will others think? Will I ever be trusted again? How much trouble am I in? Why can't I concentrate?
4: Enduring the inquisition	Realization of seriousness. Reiterate case scenario. Respond to "whys." Interact with different responders. Understanding disclosure to family. Physical/psychosomatic symptoms.	How do I document? What happens next? Who can I talk to? Will I lose my job/license? How much trouble am I in?
5: Obtaining emotional first aid	Get/receive help. Litigation concerns emerge.	Why did I respond in this manner? What is wrong with me? Do I need help? Where can I turn for help?
6: Moving on (three possible paths)	***Drop out*** Transfer. Quit. Feelings of inadequacy. ***Survive*** Cope, but with intrusive thoughts. Persistent sadness, try to learn. ***Thrive*** Maintain life/work balance. Gain insight/perspective. Advocate for patient safety.	Should I be in this profession? How could I have prevented this? Why do I still feel so badly? What can I learn from this? What can I do to make it better?

Source: Scott, S. D., Hirschinger, L. E., Cox, K. R., McCoig, M., Brandt, J., & Hall, L. W. (2009). The natural history of recovery for the healthcare provider "second victim" after adverse patient events. *Quality and Safety in Healthcare*, p. 329. doi: 10.1136/qshc.2009.032870.

identity; and uncertainties about which errors to disclose and about how to do it (Kaldjian, Jones, Rosenthal, Tripp-Reimer, & Hillis, 2006, p. 945).

Generally, a well-intentioned and grounded professional will work through the objections to disclosure and recognize that disclosure is inevitable. On signing the surrender document that ended World War II, Emperor Hirohito admonished his people ". . . to endure the unendurable and suffer what is insufferable." Disclosing an error will feel the same way to most practitioners. Practitioners who suffer from an exaggerated sense of self-importance and exhibit the additional traits of a pathological medical narcissist will likely not disclose the error. Pathological medical narcissists will

- Act in accord with an ideal self-image arising from a core of self-doubt and insecurity
- Act defensively when this ideal self-image is threatened
- Lose feelings for others as energy is devoted to defending the ideal self-image
- Exhibit a manic quest for success and achievement
- Exploit others to achieve this success and achievement
- Disown the real self that is flawed

Such individuals will attempt to rationalize or reinterpret the situation to protect themselves when disclosing the error. They will do this by using euphemistic language, distorting the consequences of the error, displacing responsibility, or making an advantageous comparison to something worse. The goal of this rationalization is for the healthcare professional to convince him- or herself that not disclosing the error, or a less than truthful disclosure, is not morally or professionally wrong.

Coping

NURSE KIMBERLY HIATT ADMINISTERED 1.4 grams of calcium chloride instead of 140 milligrams to an 8-month-old pediatric patient. Five days later the baby died. Given the baby's condition, it is not clear that the mistake killed the baby, but it clearly exacerbated the baby's cardiac dysfunction. Hiatt was fired, sanctioned by the state nursing commission, fined $3,000, required to take 80 hours of coursework on medication administration, and placed on 4 years' probation. Hiatt committed suicide by hanging at age 50. She left two children. Hiatt's mother, a former nurse, said, "She was in such anguish. She ran out of coping skills" (Aleccia, 2011).

Suicide is a form of coping, as are substance abuse, alcoholism, emotionally acting out, or any other reckless behavior following the trauma of an error. Each of these coping strategies is obviously dysfunctional. Categorizing suicide as a coping strategy is not meant to be facetious, but it is a way to eliminate the emotional pain.

Effectively coping with a medication error requires three things. First, one has to experience and work through all the emotions associated with the error. Denying or suppressing those emotions will ultimately lead to problems. Stoicism may be the ideal while at work; however, late at night in your room self-reflection is preferred. Depending on the severity of the error there is a reasonable "mourning period" following the error. For a near-miss that doesn't get to the patient, an evening after work dealing with the emotional aftermath may be sufficient. For a fatal error, a year may be in order. This period will vary for individuals; the point is that there should be a natural and healthy limit. If someone close to you has died, think of how long the recovery period was for that circumstance. At some point after the error it is incumbent to "get on with it." Having felt and analyzed the attendant emotions they need to be wrapped up and put in the emotional equivalent of the old business file. If this is not possible, and the emotions associated with the error are still too close to the surface, professional help is in order. Situational depression following an error is appropriate; prolonged depression is a disease.

Imagine making a fatal error. Now imagine standing in front of the mirror as you get ready for work. What would you be telling yourself as you gaze into the mirror? It is this self-talk that is critical to the second stage of coping with the error. Some of the things you say to yourself will be appropriate; they will be both accurate and functional. Other things you say to yourself will not be. The emotional intelligence exercise at the end of the chapter asks you to list the things you would tell yourself as you look in the mirror, and then rate their accuracy and usefulness. The one fundamental thing you cannot say to yourself and expect to successfully cope with the error is this: I made a mistake; I am a failure. This line of thinking is neither accurate nor helpful in resurrecting and continuing your career. A more appropriate line of thinking is something like this: I'm a well-meaning professional who has put hours into honing my skills. For various reasons, some of which I controlled and some of which I could not, an error was made. I did the best I could both before and after the error. I now recognize there are better ways to do things, which I will incorporate into my practice. I know of no way to practice, and continue to help people, where all possibility of error is eliminated.

In the title of his book about managing medical failure, Charles Bosk offers the final and best way to think about errors—to *Forgive and Remember*. Ultimately, you must forgive yourself. Although you are a professional, you also are human, and no human is perfect. You must remember that so the mistakes you made are never repeated and the lessons learned are applied to the patients you will help for the rest of your career.

The final step in coping with the error is a detached and systematic analysis of the error, from both a personal perspective and a systems organizational perspective. The professional requirement of excellence demands it. Generally, for a fatal error to occur multiple circumstances have to line up in such a way that the error gets through. In other words, most errors are caught due to professional expertise or redundant safeguards built into the systems. A specific error gets made, on a certain day, with a certain type of patient, with the wrong drug, and the catastrophic error occurs. If any single variable changed in this sequence, the outcomes would have been completely different. It is this analysis that will ultimately bring psychological closure to the professional. Having made this analysis, and improved their practice skills, the individual can take comfort first in meeting the professional standard, but then in understanding that the experience, as awful as it may have been, was not wasted. Although one or two people may have suffered, innumerable lives in immeasurable ways will be enhanced.

Medication Errors at Work

THE FOLLOWING IS A SAMPLE scenario related to medication errors involving RPG (recent pharmacy graduate):

RPG had never seen a table so long. Now, arrayed in front of him, was the entire state board of pharmacy. He had been called in to discuss a medication error he had made 2 years ago. A patient had been given an unusually large dose of prednisone, by mistake. RPG was responsible for misreading the directions, and typing in QID for QD. RPG explained what happened. They seemed satisfied with the explanation, at least to the extent that they believed the error was an honest mistake without overtones of complete negligence or egregious disregard. Nevertheless, they required RPG to attend 10 hours of continuing education programs over the next year.

The whole affair had been humiliating. RPG felt everyone at work was looking at him and discussing the error and his circumstances behind his back. For 6 months, RPG had been operating under a self-imposed blanket of sadness with tinges of anger and self-pity. Don't they all recognize what sacrifices I had to make to go to pharmacy school? On the way home in the car, RPG found himself sitting at a stop sign crying. He didn't move until the car behind him honked. RPG was also consuming a bottle of wine each night with dinner, rather than his customary one glass. RPG had also put on 30 pounds in the last 6 months. None of his pants fit anymore. RPG found himself puffing when walking up stairs. RPG also just found out that his wife was pregnant. Great, he thought, one more thing I can screw up.

How would you recommend RPG handle the situation?

Assignment: What Do the Practitioners/Others Say?

BE PREPARED TO DISCUSS WORRY, fear, and errors based on any *one* of the following:

- A discussion with your colleagues, or others, on how they feel and what they know about worry, fear, and errors

- An article on worry, fear, and errors, from either the research literature or any other source

- A movie/television program/YouTube video about worry, fear, and errors

- A book on worry, fear, and errors (literary, historical, psychological, or any other source)

EXERCISES

⊕ Worry Log

Over the next week keep a log of all the things you worry about and how much time you to devote to this activity.

⊕ Fear of Failure: Performance Appraisal Inventory (Short-Form)

Please answer the following questions using this response scale:

−2	−1	0	+1	+2
Do Not Believe at All		Believe 50% of the Time		Believe 100% of the Time

1. When I am failing, I am afraid that I might not have enough talent. _____

2. When I am failing, it upsets my "plan" for the future. _____

3. When I am not succeeding, people are less interested in me. _____

4. When I am failing, important others are disappointed. _____

5. When I am failing, I worry about what others might think about me. _____

ITEM (1. _____ + 2. _____ + 3. _____ + 4. _____ + 5. _____) = _____ /5 = _____

Norms for College-Age Students

Percentile	Score
95	1.342
90	1.035
85	0.831
80	0.667
75	0.527
70	0.400
65	0.284
60	0.173
55	0.066
50	−0.040
45	−0.146
40	−0.253

35	−0.364
30	−0.481
25	−0.607
20	−0.747
15	−0.911
10	−1.115
5	−1.422

Source: Conroy, D. E. (2003). *The performance failure appraisal inventory* (1st ed.). College Park, PA: Department of Kinesiology, College of Health and Human Development, The Pennsylvania State University, p. 123.

⊪ **What Exactly Is a Failure?**

Please indicate which of the following circumstances constitutes a failure. Check the ones you consider to be a failure.

1. You are the world record holder in the marathon. You come in first but miss the world record by 8 seconds. _____

2. You are a world class runner. However, you have never finished higher than 10th in this event. You finish 6th and do *not* beat your best time. _____

3. You are a world class runner. However, you have never finished higher than 10th in this event. You finish 11th and beat your best time.

4. You beat the age group (over 55) record time, but finish in the last 300 runners. _____

5. You have never run a marathon before, but finish in the last 50 runners. _____

6. You have completed one other marathon. This time you do not finish the race. _____

7. You first ran in this race 60 years ago. This year you come to the race to help with the organization. _____

Ask yourself, is it a failure if you do not get the residency you want, but get your third choice? Have to take the NAPLEX a second time? Realize after a year that community practice is not for you and go back to graduate school at a reduced salary? Get a raise but not as much as you think? Get assigned to the committee you want but are not named the chair? Is there a subjective element to failure, or is anything less than number one a failure?

⊪ Medication Errors and the Emotional Intelligence Framework

All people ultimately must confront the fact that they are not perfect; that success and failure are the fabric of life. Simultaneously, all pharmacists must ultimately confront the fact of errors. Emotional intelligence is an appropriate framework to confront these fears and anxieties.

> *Self-aware:* Imagine making a fatal error. Now imagine standing in front of the mirror as you get ready for work. What would you be telling yourself as you gaze into the mirror?

> *Self-management:* In the past, how have you managed yourself when confronted with failure, not making a team, not passing a test, being rejected? What did you do correctly, and what can be improved on?

> *Social awareness:* Think of how someone is likely to present themselves following a fatal medication error—their demeanor, their body language, their voice, and their conversations. How would you present yourself?

> *Relationship management:* How should you manage your relationship with your boss, your coworkers, the victim's family, and your family following a fatal medication error?

⊪ Personal Learning Plan: Success and Failure

These steps can be compiled on a single page containing the following:

> What prompted me to develop this plan?

> What is the general area for improvement?

> What is the specific issue for improvement?

> Why is this important to me?

> How do I generally act in these areas?

> What are my goals?

> What prompted this effort?

> What strategies are required?

> Who/what is necessary to meet my goals with this strategy?

How will I measure the success/failure of this effort?

How long will I focus on this effort?

How will I reflect and capture a lesson from this effort that can be generalized to other circumstances.

Based on your responses, write a one-paragraph description of yourself as it relates to worry, fear, and ethics.

⊕ WHAT'S IMPORTANT TO YOU IN THE CHAPTER?

With several of your classmates, discuss the idea/ideas that are most likely to effect change in your values, attitudes, or behaviors. Be succinct—no more than two sentences.

⊕ REFERENCES

Aleccia, J. (2011). Nurse's suicide highlights twin tragedies of medical errors. Retrieved from http://www.msnbc.com/id/43529641/ns/health-health_ care/t/nurses-suicide-highlights-twin-tragedies-medical errors/.

Bosk, C. L. (1979). *Forgive and remember.* Chicago, IL: University of Chicago Press.

Christensen, J. F., Levinson, W., & Dunn, P. M. (1992). The heart of darkness: The impact of perceived mistakes on physicians. *Journal of General Internal Medicine, 7,* 425–431.

Conroy, D. E. (2001). Progress in the development of a multidimensional measure of fear of failure: The performance failure appraisal inventory (PFAI). *Anxiety, Stress, and Coping, 14,* 431–452.

Conroy, D. E. (2003). *The performance failure appraisal inventory* (1st ed.). College Park, PA: Department of Kinesiology, College of Health and Human Development, The Pennsylvania State University.

Coontz, S. (2012, February 11). The M. R. S. and the Ph. D. *New York Times Sunday Review.* Retrieved from http://www.nytimes.com /2012/02/12/opinion/sunday/marriage-suits-educated-women. html?pageswanted=all.

Ekman, P., & Cordaro, D. (2011). What is meant by calling emotions basic. *Emotion Review, 3*(4), 364–370.

Institute of Medicine. (2007). *Preventing medication errors: quality chasm series.* National Academy of Sciences. Retrieved from http://books.nap.edu/catalog11623.html.

Kaiser Family Foundation (2010). Prescription Drug Trends.

Kaldjian, L. C., Jones, E. W., Rosenthal, G. E., Tripp-Reimer, T., & Hillis. S. L. (2006). An empirically derived taxonomy of factors affecting physicians' willingness to disclose medical errors. *Journal of General Internal Medicine, 21,* 942–948.

Kohn, L. T., Corrigan, J. M., & Donaldson, M. S. (2000). *To err is human.* Institute of Medicine, National Academy Press: Washington, DC. http://www.nap.edu/openbook/9728/png/R1.png.

Martin, A. J., & Marsh, H. W. (2003). Fear of failure: Friend or foe. *Australian Psychologist, 38*(1), 31–38.

McLean, C. P., & Anderson, E. R. (2009). Brave men and timid women? A review of the gender differences in fear and anxiety. *Clinical Psychology Review, 29,* 496–505.

Scott, S. D., Hirschinger, L. E., Cox, K. R., McCoig, M., Brandt, J., & Hall, L. W. (2009). The natural history of recovery for the healthcare provider "second victim" after adverse patient events. *Quality and Safety in Healthcare.* doi: 10.1136/qshc.2009.032870.

Sender, J. W., & Moray, N. P. (1991). *Human error: Cause, prediction, and reduction.* Hillsdale, NJ: Lawrence Erlbaum Associates.

Waterman, A. D., Garbutt, J., Hazel, E., et al. (2007). The emotional impact of medical errors on practicing physicians in the United States and Canada. *Joint Commission Journal of Quality and Patient Safety, 33*(8), 467–476.

Wu, A. W., Folkman, S., McPhee. S. J., et al. (1993). How house officers cope with their mistakes. *Western Journal of Medicine, 159,* 565–569.

⬥ SUGGESTED READINGS

Banja, J. (2005). *Medical errors and medical narcissism.* Boston, MA: Jones and Bartlett.

Fried-Buchalter, S. (1997). Fear of success, fear of failure, and the imposter phenomenon among male and female marketing managers. *Sex Roles, 37*(11/12), 847–859.

Janda, L. (1999). *Career tests.* Avon, MA: Adams Media.

Meron, A., Borkovec, T. D., & Ruscio, J. (2001). A taxometric investigation of the latent structure of worry. *Journal of Abnormal Psychology, 110*(3), 413–422.

Meyer, T. J., Miller, M. L., Metzger, R. L., & Borkovec, T. D. (1990). Development and validation of the Penn State Worry Questionnaire. *Behavior Research and Therapy, 28,* 487–495.

Mockler, R. J., & Dologite, D. G. (1999). Learning how to learn: Nurturing professional growth through cognitive mapping. *New England Journal of Entrepreneurship, 2*(2), 65–80.

Neenan, M. (2009). *Developing resilience.* London, UK: Routledge.

Nolen-Hoeksema, S., Morrow, J., & Frederickson, B. L. (1993). Response styles and the duration of episodes of depressed mood. *Journal of Abnormal Psychology, 102,* 20–28.

Ouiment, A. J., Gawronski, B., & Dozois, D. J. A. (2009). Cognitive vulnerability to anxiety, a review and integrative model. *Clinical Psychology Review, 29,* 459–470.

Sirriyeh, R., Lawton, R., Gardner, P., & Armitage, G. (2010). Coping with medical error: A systematic review of papers to assess the effects of involvement in medical errors on healthcare professionals' psychological well-being. *Quality and Safety in Healthcare.* doi:10.1136/qshc.2009.035253.

Wright, A. G. C., Pincus, A. L., Conroy, D. E., & Elliott, A. J. The pathoplastic relationship between interpersonal problems and fear of failure. *Journal of Personality, 77*(4), 997–1024.

Zuckerman, M., & Allison, S. N. (1976) An objective measure of fear of success: Construction and validation. *Journal of Personality Assessment, 40,* 422–430.

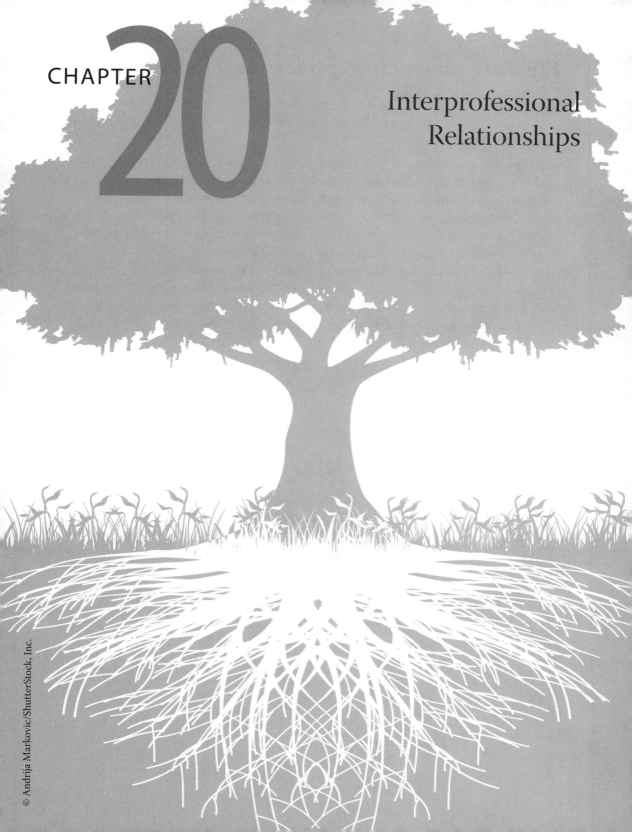

CHAPTER

20

Interprofessional
Relationships

Pre-Assessment: Interprofessional Relationships

Mind Mapping

Consider the terms arrayed on the page. For each term, without thinking or editing, write down the ideas, concepts, examples, contradictions, and theories that come to mind. Do not array them in any systematic or orderly manner. Scatter them about the page. Now, draw lines between your additions, indicating that there is a relationship between the terms. If something causes something else, indicate this with an arrow. Relationships may be reciprocal—both cause each other—requiring arrows at both ends. Indicate the strength of the relationship by darkening and thickening the lines; stronger relationships have darker and thicker lines. Most important: There is no right answer. Do not compare with your classmates. *What you have is a mind map, your mental representation of the topic. Review to determine if anything has changed following this section.*

Power at work
Relating to doctors
Relating to nurses
Relating to pharmacists
Relating to technicians

⦚ DESIRED EDUCATIONAL OUTCOMES

- Discuss the types of professional relationships.
- Discuss the bases of social power.
- Understand and discuss professional transactions.

⦚ DESIRED PERSONAL OUTCOME

- Enhance interprofessional relationships.

Introduction

GOOD WORKING RELATIONSHIPS ARE BASED on trust, respect, team-work, and open communication. Trust derives from meeting others' expectations and knowing that the other professional has integrity. Even if a colleague is not likeable, they are deserving of respect. Respect is having a colleague take your recommendation because it is you who made it, without having to verify or confirm your work. Open communication is the ability to say what needs to be said because the patient comes first, not egos. It is the ability to question and be questioned without defensiveness. Teamwork is the movement of collaboration from individual relationships to all professionals involved. Collegial relationships have all the features of a collaborative relationship with the added dimension of equality. Equality of professional relationships rests on the understanding that each discipline involved in patient care has a unique and essential perspective.

Power

CURRENT INTERPROFESSIONAL RELATIONSHIPS ARE A result of the history of each of the professions involved. For much of that history there were significant differences in power and responsibility for the various professions. Variance in this power resulted in institutional subservience and dominance. Interprofessional power, as well as all social power, rests on five bases. Those power bases are (French & Raven, 1959):

- *Coercive power:* The ability to force someone to do something they don't want to do; the goal is compliance. This type of power relies on threats and punishment.

Box 20.1   Types of Professional Relationships

Five types of professional relationships are presented here in descending order of impact on patient outcomes:

- ❑ *Collegial:* Equal power, trust, and respect
- ❑ *Collaborative:* Mutual power, trust, and respect
- ❑ *Student–teacher:* Either party can be the student or teacher; both parties are willing to listen, teach, and learn
- ❑ *Friendly stranger:* Little trust and acknowledgement; may be courteous but formal
- ❑ *Hostile, adversarial, and abusive:* Negativity in tone and action

Professional relationships are subject to change. Moving from being friendly strangers to a student–teacher relationship is an enhancement. Devolving to a hostile relationship is obviously not. Even these relationships can be rehabilitated, however. Collaborative relationships reflect working together, sharing responsibilities for solving problems, and making plans for patient care.

Source: Adapted from Schmalenberg, C., Kramer, M., King, C. R., Krugman, M., Lund, C., Poduska, D., & Rapp, D. (2005). Securing collegial/collaborative nurse–physician relationships, part 1. *Journal of Nursing Administration*, 35(10), 451.

- • *Reward power:* The ability to provide someone with something they want, or remove something they don't want. Raises, promotions, and compliments typify this type of power. In an academic context, grades are used to reward behavior.

- • *Legitimate power:* Stems from the position one occupies. A director of pharmacy has legitimate power.

- • *Referent power:* This is power derived from respect for another person, someone who is exceptionally good at their job.

- • *Expert power:* This is power derived from the information, knowledge, or expertise that an individual has. It is derived from being a leading expert.

One person may combine all of the bases of social power, though it is not likely. In dealing with other professionals it is critical to understand the bases of their power. A residency director may have legitimate power but very little expert power, having been off the floor for several years. In handling professional relationships, a key is an understanding of the power differences and the sources of power. Relating to a world-class transplant surgeon is completely different from how you would relate to a student intern.

Professional Transactions

ONE METHOD OF CONSIDERING PROFESSIONAL relationships is to examine the nature and types of transactions between professionals. First, consider the perspectives individuals might adopt when interacting with one another.

Consummate professional: A consummate professional's sole focus is the patient and their well-being. Acting as a consummate professional involves considering the situation and the available information in an objective, unbiased manner, to arrive at unprejudiced conclusions. In a clinical situation, acting as the consummate professional involves considering: Is the information valid? Does the information apply in this case? Are clinical decisions appropriate from a clinical, ethical, and financial perspective? Personal issues and agendas, ego, insecurities, politics, and emotional distortions are absent when acting as consummate professionals. Consummate professionals are in control of themselves and recognize they are *only* in control of themselves, not any other professional. A student can act as a consummate professional by understanding their obligations and responsibilities in a given circumstance.

Professor/boss: Acting as the professor/boss means to act based on the idea of "should" and "ought"—that there are standards that need not be examined for validity and appropriateness and are invoked in an unthinking manner. The professor/boss thinks: This is the way it is done, why don't you know this? The professor/boss may say one thing and do something else. In other words, they are willing to impose standards on you, but cut corners for themselves. Much of what the professor/boss believes is appropriate. These well-structured and strongly held beliefs expedite outcomes. The professor/boss is never in doubt. They believe they are in control of everything. Any problems that arise in a professional relationship are your fault.

Student/employee: There are two aspects to the student/employee perspective. The first is inappropriate and may be dysfunctional. The student/employee believes they are not responsible for anything, not even themselves. Their fallback attitude is: I was just following the rules, the protocols, what you told me. The student/employee tends to blame others for outcomes and takes no responsibility for the consequences of their actions. The second perspective is positive. In this case, the student/employee is engaged in understanding how they might improve. They willingly defer to expertise in any form to facilitate improved patient outcomes. Even the 40-year practitioner committed to excellence will, at times, adopt this perspective.

All professionals exhibit aspects of each perspective over the course of their professional lives. In fact, they may exhibit each perspective in a single transaction. The key is to understand when each is appropriate. The ideal professional transaction obviously involves two consummate professionals acting with equal power and trust in a collegial relationship to positively impact patient outcomes based on objective criteria. In certain professional transactions a professor/boss and student/employee is more than appropriate; it is desired. One of the professionals may, in fact, be a student/employee, but it is also possible that a consummate professional adopts a student/employee perspective for a specific transaction where appropriate. Problems arise when both professionals want to act as the professor/boss; when each wants to avoid responsibility and act as the student/employee; and when one party acts as the professor/boss and the other as the consummate professional. Long-term interprofessional issues arise if one always acts out of the professor/boss or student/employee mode. The point of this framework is to provide a method of analysis and a guide for productive and nonproductive interprofessional relationships.

The framework just described borrows from the work of Berne (*Games People Play*, 1964) and Harris (*I'm OK—You're OK*, 1969). In their works, transactions are analyzed from the perspective of the parent (professor/boss), the adult (consummate professional), and the child (student/employee). In any professional transaction think of who is acting like the critical, controlling parent; the functioning, objective adult; and the passive, weak child.

It is important to understand that all interprofessional relationships have two aspects—the observable social aspect and the psychological aspect. The relationship may appear to be between two consummate professionals, but what is actually going on is an unspoken, and often little understood, attempt to avoid responsibility (student/employee), assert dominance (professor/boss), or defend egos (both). The point is that relationships always have a subtext that may or may not conform to what is actually said and observed. The adherence to a strict protocol by the professor/boss may be an attempt to avoid responsibility, and the powerlessness of a student/employee may be a ploy to maintain control and get someone else to do the work.

Interprofessional Relationships at Work

THE FOLLOWING ARE SAMPLE SCENARIOS related to interprofessional relationships involving RPG (recent pharmacy graduate):

Pharmacists

The hospital was not for the faint of heart. It was high volume and high pressure. It was the lead teaching hospital in a major health system. World class physicians, procedures, and research characterized the environment. If you didn't know your business you would soon be found out. The place was known for the rapid turnover of pharmacy staff. In the hospital there was a core group of pharmacists that had survived and prospered in this environment. Like soldiers on a battlefield who didn't bother to learn the new recruits' names because they would soon be dead, support for a new pharmacist from the core group was nonexistent. In fact, it was almost antagonistic. RPG watched how the latest new hire was being treated and wondered whether the hospital or the other pharmacists were the cause of the turnover.

How would you recommend RPG handle the situation?

Nurses

RPG did just about everything she could to avoid one of the nurses on the floor. The nurse was exceedingly difficult to work with. She knew her business, but was often curt and overly blunt, as if she had little time for small talk or foolishness. One afternoon RPG and the nurse got into it on the floor over a small matter. RPG was considering going to the nursing supervisor with a complaint, but wanted to think about it over the weekend.

How would you recommend RPG handle the situation?

Physicians

The physician was almost a caricature of the kindly old family physician. He was kind-hearted but could, at best, be said to practice 1960s medicine. In the small rural hospital where RPG was director, the physician was universally loved by the patients, the staff, and the community. Lately RPG had noticed that the physician's drug protocols were moving from dated to possibly harmful. At lunch one day, the hospital administrator asked for RPG's assessment of the drug regimens the physician utilized. Although those protocols were inexpensive due to the number of older medications utilized, the administrator had noticed that outcome data for the hospital was declining.

How would you recommend RPG handle the situation?

Technicians

RPG watched as one of his colleague pharmacists yelled at the technician about a mistake. It was more than a conversation about something gone wrong. The pharmacist was demeaning the technician. RPG understood that sometimes the technicians tended to exceed their authority, but she also recognized they were crucial to the operation of the pharmacy because they filled most of the orders and parenterals. RPG wondered if her colleagues saw technicians as professionals, and what the appropriate relationship with technicians should be.

How would you recommend RPG handle the situation?

Assignment: What Do the Practitioners/ Others Say?

B E PREPARED TO DISCUSS INTERPROFESSIONAL relationships based on any *one* of the following:

- A discussion with your colleagues, or others, on how they feel and what they know about interprofessional relationships

- An article on interprofessional relationships, from either the research literature or any other source

- A movie/television program/YouTube video on interprofessional relationships

- A book on interprofessional relationships (literary, historical, psychological, or any other source)

EXERCISES

1. In dealing with a student intern, characterize an appropriate professional relationship. What is appropriate if the student intern is not performing at an adequate clinical level? If the intern is performing at an adequate professional level?

2. What would you conclude about an individual who was rude to wait-staff in a restaurant? Would you want to work with such a person?

Based on your responses, write a one-paragraph description of yourself as it relates to interprofessional relationships.

Interprofessional Relationships and the Emotional Intelligence Framework

Using the professor/boss–consummate professional–student/employee framework described earlier in the chapter, consider the following:

Self-aware: Which perspective do you typically adopt when dealing with other professionals? Other students on projects?

Self-management: Can you shift from one perspective to another where appropriate?

Social awareness: Characterize the students in your closest circle of acquaintances using the framework. Do the same for the professionals you associate with at work.

Relationship management: Speculate if there is a subtext to the most difficult relationships you have at work.

ⅰ Personal Learning Plan: Interprofessional Relationships

These steps can be compiled on a single page containing the following:

What prompted me to develop this plan?

What is the general area for improvement?

What is the specific issue for improvement?

Why is this important to me?

How do I generally act in these areas?

What are my goals?

What prompted this effort?

What strategies are required?

Who/what is necessary to meet my goals with this strategy?

How will I measure the success/failure of this effort?

How long will I focus on this effort?

How will I reflect and capture a lesson from this effort that can be generalized to other circumstances.

ⅰ WHAT'S IMPORTANT TO YOU IN THE CHAPTER?

With several of your classmates, discuss the idea/ideas that are most likely to effect change in your values, attitudes, or behaviors. Be succinct—no more than two sentences.

ⅰ REFERENCES

Berne, E. (1964). *Games people play*. New York, NY: Ballantine.

French, J. R. P., & Raven, B. H. (1959). *The bases of social power*. In D. Cartwright (ed.) *Studies in social power* (pp. 150–167). Ann Arbor, MI: Institute for Social Research.

Harris, T. A. (1969). *I'm OK—you're OK*. New York, NY: Harper.

Schmalenberg, C., Kramer, M., King, C. R., Krugman, M., Lund, C., Poduska, D., & Rapp, D. (2005). Securing collegial/collaborative nurse–physician relationships, part 1. *Journal of Nursing Administration*, *35*(10), 450–458.

⑩ SUGGESTED READINGS

Fostering the pharmacist-physician relationship. (2009). *American Journal of Health-System Pharmacy*, *66*, 118–119.

Hawk, C., Buckwalter, K., Byrd, L., Cigelman, S., Dorfman, L., & Ferguson, K. (2002). Health professions students' perceptions of interprofessional relationships. *Academic Medicine*, *77*(4), 354–357.

Kececi, A., & Tasocak, G. (2009). Nurse faculty members' ego states: Transactional analysis approach. *Nurse Education Today*, *29*, 746–752.

Lawrence, L. (2007). Applying transactional analysis and personality assessment to improve patient counseling and communication skills. *American Journal of Pharmaceutical Education*, *71*(4), 1–5.

McMahan, E. M., Hoffman, K., & McGee, G. W. (1994). Physician–nurse relationships in clinical setting: A review and critique of the literature, 1966–1992. *Medical Care Research and Review*, *51*, 83–112.

Mockler, R. J., & Dologite, D. G. (1999). Learning how to learn: Nurturing professional growth through cognitive mapping. *New England Journal of Entrepreneurship*, *2*(2), 65–80.

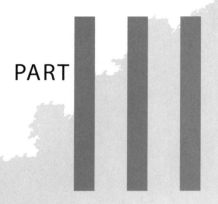

PART III

Commandments for Clinical Responsibility

At the end of each chapter you were asked to list what was important to you in that chapter. Collect the statements for each chapter and review. Can any statements be combined, eliminated, or synthesized into simpler and more personally useful statements? The task is to arrive at the fewest statements that capture the essence of what is important and memorable. In other words, what are you likely to remember in 6 months or a year? Consult with your classmates on this exercise.

⫸ WHAT'S IMPORTANT TO YOU IN THE CHAPTER?

Expertise and Thinking:

Emotional Labor, Compassion Fatigue, Stress, and Burnout:

Establishing Credibility:

Worry, Fear, and Errors:

Interprofessional Relationships:

IV

Work

Without question, pharmacy is a profession with increasing clinical responsibilities. Very few practitioners operate in a vacuum removed from the daily struggles and irritations of organizational life. Pharmacy is a job. Students are not born understanding the rules of organizational life. Although you may have a good head start on how to prosper and function at work, based on jobs you held while in school, the game changes once you become a fully vested participant following graduation and licensure.

An understanding of how careers progress, the problems of a new supervisor, how to conduct a difficult conversation, how to deal with your boss, how to survive office politics, how to handle romantic relationships, who to trust, and how to delegate and empower employees is not only helpful, but required. A practitioner that doesn't understand work will not be a practitioner for long.

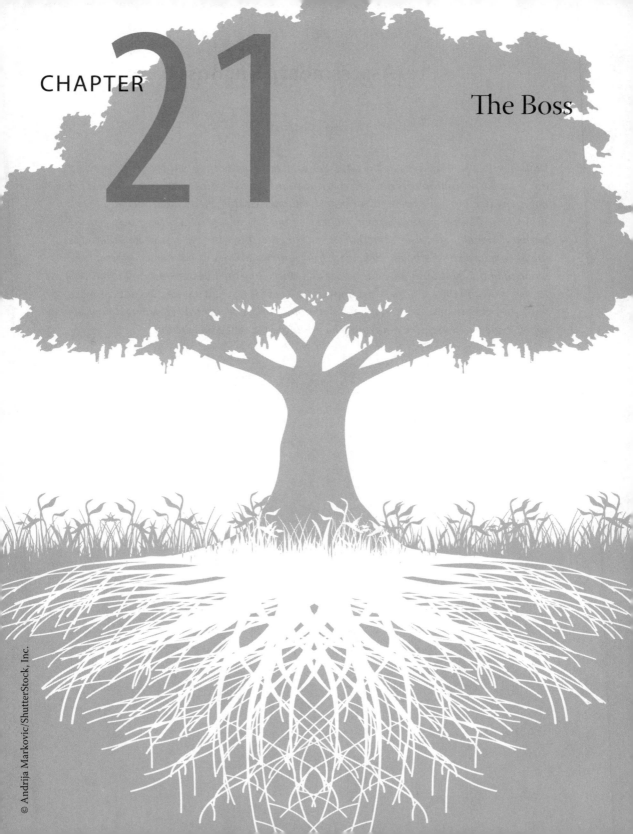

CHAPTER

21

The Boss

Pre-Assessment: The Boss

Mind Mapping

Consider the terms arrayed on the page. For each term, without thinking or editing, write down the ideas, concepts, examples, contradictions, and theories that come to mind. Do not array them in any systematic or orderly manner. Scatter them about the page. Now, draw lines between your additions, indicating that there is a relationship between the terms. If something causes something else, indicate this with an arrow. Relationships may be reciprocal—both cause each other—requiring arrows at both ends. Indicate the strength of the relationship by darkening and thickening the lines; stronger relationships have darker and thicker lines. Most important: There is no right answer. Do not compare with your classmates. *What you have is a mind map, your mental representation of the topic. Review to determine if anything has changed following this section.*

Best boss you worked for
Worst boss you worked for

⚜ **DESIRED EDUCATIONAL OUTCOMES**

- Describe the assumptions in managing your boss.
- Discuss how to shape your boss's behavior.

⚜ **DESIRED PERSONAL OUTCOME**

- Improve your relationship with your boss.

What Are the Key Assumptions to Managing Your Boss?

THE SINGLE GREATEST REASON WHY people leave a job is their relationship with their boss. The key relationship one has at work, without exception, is with the boss. This single individual in many ways determines the path and trajectory of your career. Hit it off with the boss and that path is facilitated; be unfortunate enough to clash with your boss and many doors close.

You don't have to like or admire your boss, you do have to manage him or her for career advancement.

Certain key assumptions are useful in the process of managing your boss:

- You own 50% of your relationship with your boss.
- You are 100% in control of your own behavior.
- The way you behave toward your boss teaches him or her how to treat you.
- The relationship with your boss is one of mutual dependence.
- You are both fallible human beings.

Who Is Dependent on Whom?

SOME PEOPLE SEE THEMSELVES AS extremely dependent on their boss. As such, they adopt an infantile posture toward their boss. They see their boss as omnipotent and infallible. In fact, the boss is insecure and uncertain, as are all humans. One needs to recognize just how dependent the boss is on his or her subordinates. Through your actions you can do him or her considerable harm. Bosses are imperfect. They are fallible. They don't have all the answers. Nor are they the enemy.

What Do I Need to Understand?

MANAGING YOUR BOSS REQUIRES THAT you understand your boss, the context in which he or she operates, and his or her pressures, goals, strengths, and weaknesses. What does your boss do well? What is his or her style of working, of communicating? Does he or she like conflict or avoid it? Does he or she have any personal idiosyncrasies? You must recognize that your boss is not likely to change, and that you are not likely to change him or her.

Similarly, you need to be candid in assessing yourself. What are your strengths and weaknesses? What are your goals and objectives? How do you prefer to communicate? And do you have any idiosyncrasies? In looking for points of resonance between you and your boss, the following questions are helpful:

- What are your boss's three greatest strengths/weaknesses? What are my three greatest strengths/weaknesses?
- What things do we work on effectively together?
- What are our greatest sources of conflict and disagreement?
- What is the weakest aspect of our relationship?

Understanding your boss's strengths and weaknesses, as well as your own, is the foundation for crafting a positive relationship with your boss. First, if his or her preferred work style is one of formal communication via memos and reports, then you should adjust your behavior to that style—whether you like it or not. Second, mutual expectations for one another should be explicitly declared. Typically, your boss won't do this and it is your job to solicit this information. Third, keep a flow of information moving upward toward him or her. You may need to find a way to frame information that he or she doesn't want, such as failures and problems. Fourth, be dependable and honest in dealing with your boss. It is the only way he or she will learn to trust you and confide in you. Fifth, be judicious in your demands on his or her time.

Can I Shape My Boss's Behavior?

ALTHOUGH YOU CAN'T CHANGE YOUR boss's behavior, you can shape it. For example, if you would like him or her to speak more tactfully to you in public, then every time he or she behaves in the way you like, reward him or her; for example, after the kind of encounter you want say something like, "I really appreciate how this meeting went. It reaffirms why I like working here." The list of benefits you can provide your boss as an employee are limited. Remember, bosses are human. They want affirmation, strokes, and compliments like everyone else. So, in shaping your boss's behavior keep the following in mind:

- Bosses like praise for their good points, just like everyone else.
- Voice public and private support for their goals.
- Simplify their job by taking on tasks that speak to your strengths and compensate for their weaknesses.
- Offer to be a sounding board for their ideas and problems.
- Let people know that you are proud to work for him or her.

No matter what, you will have some type of relationship with your boss. The key to a successful career is to manage that relationship. As with all relationships, a successful relationship with your boss is based on mutual understanding, respect, and benefit.

Bad Bosses

MOST OF THE BOSSES YOU will encounter will be reasonable people with varying degrees of experience, aptitude, and insight about their job. Like all people they will have bad days, display uncalled-for insensitivity, and make mistakes. Despite this they are well-meaning people, like you, trying to do the best they can. It is likely that most of the people you work for will subscribe to theories of management based on fairness and employee participation. For some bosses, however, this will not be true. Some bosses may rely on fear, intimidation, anger, and rage to motivate people. They may trample on people's feelings and set impossible standards. How do you deal with such a boss? Suggestions include the following:

- Always be prepared for meetings.
- Work harder to demonstrate your commitment.
- Demonstrate that you are not a pushover by calling their bluff in a nonconfrontational manner.
- Keep things in perspective; don't take them too seriously.
- Stick around—the longer you stay the more they will trust you.

A great response to a boss going into a rant is, "You seem upset. Why don't we talk later when things calm down?" The reason to tolerate such behavior from him or her is what working with this person can do for your career. As long as the relationship and the circumstance advance your career goals, then tolerating the situation makes sense. If not, leaving is in order.

Telling the Boss You Made a Mistake

IF YOU MAKE A MISTAKE, the best approach is to let the boss know before he or she finds out some other way. Specifically, tell him or her what happened and what your reasoning was for handling the situation the way you did. Point out the flaw in your logic or assumptions and what you learned from the situation. The key point is to convey how you fixed the problem, what the outcome was, and how you guaranteed that it wouldn't happen again. This approach speaks to your integrity regarding mistakes, your ability to act independently, and your recognition that the problem was yours, not one you expected your boss to fix.

Managing Your Boss at Work

THE FOLLOWING IS A SAMPLE scenario related to managing your boss involving RPG (recent pharmacy graduate):

Periodically, when things were slow, the pharmacist in charge would spend a few moments chatting with the staff. The pharmacist in charge had a good sense of humor, but occasionally he told a joke that was slightly off color. Though not prudish, RPG just didn't like this type of humor. She really wasn't offended by the jokes, just a little uneasy. RPG wasn't sure if she should talk to the pharmacist in charge about this because she appreciated the few moments of camaraderie with the staff. She thought the pharmacist in charge might stop the spontaneous sessions with the staff, particularly if he was embarrassed that he might have made someone uncomfortable. Instead of talking directly to the pharmacist in charge, RPG made it a point to convey to him how much she enjoyed the session, but only when he had not told a joke. She also started to tease the pharmacist in charge about how bad the jokes were. In short, she was going to try to reinforce the behavior she wanted.

How would you recommend RPG handle the situation?

Assignment: What Do the Practitioners/ Others Say?

B E PREPARED TO DISCUSS BOSSES based on any *one* of the following:

- A discussion with your boss on aspects of his or her job
- An article on bosses, from either the research literature or any other source
- A movie/television program/YouTube video about bosses
- A book on bosses (literary, historical, psychological, or any other source)

EXERCISES

1. While at work, ask your boss what he or she worries about the most. What is the hardest part of his or her job? What was the hardest thing for him or her to learn after taking the job? What was his or her strongest feeling/emotion upon accepting the position?

2. With your classmates, and based on your mind mapping exercise at the beginning of the chapter, discuss the attributes of a good boss and

a bad boss. Arrive at a consensus for these traits. For this list of traits (both good and bad), rate yourself. If you are deficient in a good trait, or possess a bad trait to a significant degree, discuss how you might deal with these deficiencies.

Based on your responses, write a one-paragraph description of yourself as a potential boss. Would you want to work for yourself?

⚬ Your Boss and the Emotional Intelligence Framework

A successful relationship with your boss is essential to a good work environment and advancing your career.

Self-aware: What feelings do you have about your boss? Does your mood change when he or she arrives?

Self-management: What tactics do you use to manage these feelings?

Social awareness: Try to look at your boss with fresh eyes. What do you think is the primary motive for his or her behavior?

Relationship management: Consider a relationship with a boss that was difficult. What did you do to correct it? Was it successful?

⚬ Personal Learning Plan: Your Boss

These steps can be compiled on a single page containing the following:

What prompted me to develop this plan?

What is the general area for improvement?

What is the specific issue for improvement?

Why is this important to me?

How do I generally act in these areas?

What are my goals?

What prompted this effort?

What strategies are required?

Who/what is necessary to meet my goals with this strategy?

How will I measure the success/failure of this effort?

How long will I focus on this effort?

How will I reflect and capture a lesson from this effort that can be generalized to other circumstances?

⚜ WHAT'S IMPORTANT TO YOU IN THE CHAPTER?

With several of your classmates, discuss the idea/ideas that are most likely to effect change in your values, attitudes, or behaviors. Be succinct—no more than two sentences.

⚜ SUGGESTED READINGS

Gabarro, J. J., & Kotter, J. J. (2005, January). Managing your boss. *Harvard Business Review*, 92–99.

Hill, L. A., & Lineback, K. (2011, January–February). Are you a good boss—or a great one? *Harvard Business Review*, 125–131.

Kramer, R. M. (2006, February). The great intimidators. *Harvard Business Review*, 88–96.

LeBoeuf, M. (1985). *Getting results.* New York, NY: Berkley.

Namie, G., & Namie, R. (2009). *The bully at work.* Naperville, IL: SourceBooks.

Scott, G. G. (2006). *A survival guide for working with bad bosses.* New York, NY: American Management Association.

Silverman, D. (2009, September). Surviving the boss from hell. *Harvard Business Review*, 33–40.

Sutton, R. I. (2010). *Good boss, bad boss.* New York, NY: Business Plus.

22

Careers

Pre-Assessment: Careers

Mind Mapping

Consider the terms arrayed on the page. For each term, without thinking or editing, write down the ideas, concepts, examples, contradictions, and theories that come to mind. Do not array them in any systematic or orderly manner. Scatter them about the page. Now, draw lines between your additions, indicating that there is a relationship between the terms. If something causes something else, indicate this with an arrow. Relationships may be reciprocal—both cause each other—requiring arrows at both ends. Indicate the strength of the relationship by darkening and thickening the lines; stronger relationships have darker and thicker lines. Most important: There is no right answer. Do not compare with your classmates. *What you have is a mind map, your mental representation of the topic. Review to determine if anything has changed following this section.*

Career
Community practice
Residency
Hospital

⸙ DESIRED EDUCATIONAL OUTCOMES

- Describe the work relationship.
- Explain what to expect during career stages.
- Describe the mentor relationship.
- Understand how to reach one's potential.
- Describe career barriers.
- Know when and how to change jobs.
- Describe the feedback process.

⸙ DESIRED PERSONAL OUTCOME

- Achieve a better career fit and enhanced career management.

What Should I Get from Work?

WORK IS AN EXCHANGE. THE reason you are employed and the justification for your salary is the fact that you add economic value in excess of the cost of your salary. You are there to solve problems for the company. You are neither entitled to nor guaranteed a job or a successful career. The only job security is in efficiently and effectively meeting the demands of the consumer marketplace. Despite what you might think, everyone in the company has this same standard to meet; everyone from the CEO to housekeeping is in the consumer satisfaction business. As Sam Walton noted, "There is only one boss. The customer. And he can fire everybody in the company from the chairman on down, simply by spending his money somewhere else." The same discipline holds for all pharmacy practice sites. Make no mistake, the company will cut your hours, close your department, or close your store if the economics warrant. Mark Twain captured this perspective by declaring, "Don't go around saying the world owes you a living; the world owes you nothing; it was here first."

Given an understanding of this reality, your part of the work exchange is to get what you want from the company; it is how you define winning the work game. Do not feel guilty about this. Your aspiration may be to rise to the upper echelons of the organization by age 40; have a stable job in a store close to your family; or go part time in 5–10 years while you raise your family. Your objective is yours alone. If a specific practice setting or organization won't let you accomplish your goals, then it is time to move.

What Should I Expect in My Career?

ALL CAREERS PROGRESS THROUGH STAGES. The concerns of a just-graduated student differ from those of a seasoned practitioner, which differ from those of a practitioner considering retirement. The early stages of a career are a period of exploration. The objective is to find a situation that fits, establish a professional identity, develop relationships, and set oneself up to succeed. The early stages of a career are for the establishment of a dream. Typically, one establishes a family in this stage. The middle stages of a career are characterized by a commitment to a specific organization, efforts to stabilize one's position, and the pursuit of responsibility, advancement, and promotion. A well-established beginning may lead to a continued upward trajectory of advancement. Balancing family and work at this stage is a challenge. Alternatively, this stage may lead to a period of maintenance of the status quo or a decline toward career regression and stagnation. Most careers end with a period of decline or disengagement as responsibilities diminish leading to a final retirement. The expectations early in a career are for uncertainty, trial, error, and self-discovery. By about age 30, a well-managed career should be positioned to take off.

What About a Mentor?

A KEY RELATIONSHIP WITH EXTENSIVE CAREER implications for any new practitioner is that of finding and connecting with a mentor. For new practitioners, mentors are the link to the organization and to the upper levels of management. A favorable word from a mentor eases the transition to greater responsibility and future promotions. In selecting a mentor, a few key points are worth remembering (adapted from Bushardt, Moore, & Debnath, 1982):

- A mentor should be someone who can help you. They need the respect of the organization and those in charge. The mentor needs to understand the formal organization and the informal relationships that govern much of work life. They need to have the knowledge and experience of how to be successful. They need the power to push for you.

- The mentor should be someone you trust. Generally, mentors are similar to the people they mentor. They should have the same values. Ideally, they should see you as a younger version of themselves.

- Mentor relationships are two-way streets. Just as the mentor helps you, remember that you have to help the mentor with their career.

- Mentors should have a successful track record with other protégés in furthering their careers. In other words, an experienced mentor is a more prized relationship than one with a first-time mentor.

A key stage in the mentor relationship is that of separation when the balance of power and need shifts. Ultimately, new practitioners move to a more equal peer relationship with the senior member. Such separations may beget misunderstanding and resentment, particularly from the senior member. You need to be conscious of this change and continue to express appreciation for all that was done to support you.

How to Reach My Potential

REACHING YOUR POTENTIAL REQUIRES INTROSPECTION and certain proactive behaviors—but it starts with a basic philosophy, or "rules of the road" (adapted from Kaplan, 2008):

- Managing your career is 100 percent your responsibility; you must act accordingly. Many promising professionals expect their superiors to mentor them, give them thoughtful coaching, provide them with challenging opportunities, and generally steer their development. Such a passive approach is likely to derail you at some point. Although your superiors will play a role, your career is your own.

- Be wary of conventional wisdom. It's almost always wrong—for you. Hopping on the bandwagon may feel good initially, but often leads to painful regrets years later. To reach your potential you must filter out peer pressure and popular opinion; assess your own passions, skills, and convictions; and then be courageous enough to act on them.

- Have faith that, although justice may not prevail at any given point in time, it should generally prevail over time. When you do suffer an injustice, you need to be willing to step back and objectively assess your own role in these events. That mind set will help you learn from inevitable setbacks and eventually bounce back. It will also help you stay focused on issues you can control as well as bolster your determination to act like the ultimate decision maker. In short, the best career advice is the rather simple statement—do what you want.

What Are Career Barriers?

VERY SELDOM IS THERE A career that is devoid of interruptions or unimpeded by career barriers. Career barriers are the brick walls that get in the way of fulfilling your career aspirations. Career barriers include getting fired, being downsized out, conflict with a supervisor, a work environment that is an ill fit, unmanageable job stress, family circumstances, and the like. Some career barriers are permanent, such as being passed over for a promotion or getting fired. Other barriers are temporary. All one has to do is wait things out because supervisors may leave and family situations change.

A key skill is to understand how to manage these barriers. The first step is to understand the likely set of emotions associated with a career setback (adapted from London, 1998):

- *Anger:* Blaming others for wronging you
- *Guilt:* Blaming oneself for this situation
- *Anxiety:* Seeing the career barrier as a threat you will not be able to handle
- *Sadness/resignation:* A sense of loss for something that is gone
- *Harm:* Feeling helpless to do something about it and you will be hurt
- *Optimism:* Hope that this challenge will work out
- *Relevance:* Understanding that something important is happening here that you need to attend to
- *Relief:* An uncomfortable and unwinnable situation is finally concluded

In addition to the emotional aspect of a career barrier, a more cognitive, dispassionate appraisal is in order. In doing so, ask the following questions (London, 1998):

- How important was the situation and the event to you?
- To what extent were you responsible for the situation and the event?
- To what extent were others responsible for the situation and the event?
- How did you want the situation to turn out?

This approach to a career barrier is essentially thinking of the situation as a case to be analyzed for what went wrong and why.

When to Change Jobs

THE FACT THAT RELATIONSHIPS END does not mean they weren't successful. Sometimes in a career a change needs to be made. How to know when such a change is warranted? When the passion to take care of the patient, consult with peers, and improve the organization is no longer there, it is time to consider a change. The specific indicators of a time to change jobs or careers include the following:

- *Feeling trapped:* When a job that was once fulfilling becomes less meaningful, when you can find no purpose in work, and you begin to look for excuses to take off
- *Feeling bored:* When you cannot generate enthusiasm for the job or no longer look forward to the challenge, but see a long pattern of monotony into the future
- *Feeling alienated:* When you sense you are not the person you want to be, when the compromises you make to fit in are gradually eroding your sense of self
- *Feeling compromised:* When the direction of the company mandates that you begin to shave corners or compromise care in a way that conflicts with your internal standards

If you find the phrase "I hate my job" running through your mind more than the casual refrain that we all periodically play and the joy is gone from work and living—a job change is probably warranted.

How to Change Jobs

CHANGING JOBS, GOING FROM AN environment that you know to the uncertainty of a job search and entrance into a new circumstance, is frightening. It is also risky. Common missteps to avoid are:

- *Not doing enough research:* Many people will devote considerable energy to buying a car, but change jobs with little due diligence. Among other things, consider the current job market, the financial stability of the company, the room for growth, the corporate culture, and who you will be working with directly. Remember, recruiters may not lie, but like all salespeople they will present their situation in the most favorable light.

- *Don't leave for money:* An extra few dollars won't compensate for a new situation that turns out to be worse than the one you just left.

- *Going "from" a job rather than "to" a job:* It is better to wait for the right situation than to bolt from a current position and then have to repeat the process all over again.

- *Taking a short-term perspective:* Careers last 50 years. Keep in mind how the decision to change jobs will play out over the long term.

If you do make a job change and it doesn't work out, then cut your losses and move on. When asked what he would do if he made a bad decision, President Truman replied that he would make another one and correct it. If changing jobs is warranted, then be strategic about it; make sure the change promotes your long-term aspirations.

If you decide to leave, how you handle the exit is important. This is not a time to settle old scores or seek repair for old wounds. The situation is what it is. Though you may be angry or hurt as a result of your experience with the company, a strategic perspective on this process mandates that you think of the next job, or the one after that. You never know who you will meet again from this company, or what their position might be. Civility and courtesy in these situations will mark you as a consummate professional, someone others will want to work with. Don't post anything in anger on the Internet that is derogatory. In short, don't burn any bridges in exiting.

How to Take Feedback

THE BEST CAREERS ARE BASED not on being perfect, but on learning the required lessons fastest and with the lowest cost following mistakes. Feedback in any form is often painful. Many people are afraid of meetings where they are most likely to have an inadequacy or deficiency highlighted. Such events often evoke fear, anxiety, hurt, sadness, ambivalence, or resignation. Such emotions often lead to acting out, denial, brooding, defensiveness, and resistance to change, all of which are detrimental to a career. The winning approach is to reframe the entire feedback process so that it is to your advantage. Feedback situations are the beginning of opportunities to improve. They are, in fact, a signal of the organization's continued interest in you and your career. Over time, life will teach you the lessons you need to know. You can choose to be proactive in response to the information coming your way both formally and informally on a daily basis, or you can choose to ignore this information and most likely receive the same message at a later date and at a higher cost. Think of feedback this way: Would you want someone to tell you of an embarrassing stain on the back of your clothes, or let you walk around all day not knowing?

The Best Career Advice

IT SEEMS STRANGE THAT AFTER almost 6 years of school and significant expense many students are still uncertain about their career and the path they should pursue. Students may wrestle with the offer of a sign-on bonus, seeking a residency, an offer to return to their hometown, or the lure of a career outside of pharmacy. This choice is a pivotal decision in one's career and one's life. The best career advice is—do what you want. Don't take a job just for the money. Don't try to please family or a fiancé. A 50-year career at 40 hours per week equates to approximately 100,000 hours spent in an activity. One hundred thousand hours of doing something you don't like, or aren't suited for, is a recipe for misery. In the end, the advice is always—do what you want. Given the pressures of student debt, money is likely to be a significant factor in a career decision. Keep in mind what the author Neil Gaiman says about this, "Nothing I ever did where the only reason for doing it was the money was ever worth it, except as bitter experience. Usually, I didn't wind up getting the money, either" (Perez-Pena, 2012).

Emotional Intelligence and Careers

THE FOLLOWING IS A SAMPLE scenario related to RPG's (recent pharmacy graduate's) career:

> RPG found herself in her last semester torn between two career options. One was to accept a sign-on bonus and go with one of the big chains. The second was to pursue a residency, most likely with the idea of a second specialized residency. Two issues confounded this choice for RPG: one, she had incurred significant debt in going to school, and two, her car had just broken down for the third time this year. Clearly, it was time to think about replacing it. The diminished salary of the residency would make replacing the car difficult. RPG thought back to her rotations and how she did not particularly enjoy the community rotations, and if she were honest with herself she knew she was not that good at processing huge numbers of orders. Sometimes she found the patients' questions in this context trivial. In contrast, RPG had loved her rotation at a women's hospital, particularly the time in the NIC unit. Her heart just went out to the babies and their families. She loved the staff. Though she felt it, RPG did not mind the stress of working with such critically ill children. At the end of the day she was drained, but strangely energized in some way she couldn't quite articulate. On her way home one night, daydreaming at the stoplight, RPG could see herself in 10 years as a board-certified pediatric specialist in a major medical center. It seemed RPG had no choice but to pursue the residency—if she wanted to be happy. Besides, she would only be 26 when she finished—plenty of time to retire the student loan debt—and a two-year lease on a new, small car would get her through.

How would you recommend RPG handle the situation?

Assignment: What Do the Practitioners/ Others Say?

BE PREPARED TO DISCUSS CAREERS based on any *one* of the following:

- A discussion with your colleagues on how they feel about their careers
- An article on careers, from either the research literature or any other source

- A movie/television program/YouTube video about careers
- A book on careers (literary, historical, psychological, or any other source)

 EXERCISES

〽 **Your Perfect Day**

Take a moment and describe your perfect day as it relates to work. What would you be doing? How would you feel at the end of each day? What career path would you be on? Would you feel more pride in announcing to your friends what you were doing than what you feel now? Would you advise a younger brother or sister to follow your career path?

〽 **Is Your Job a Good Fit?**

Take a few moments and consider the following:

1. What are you best at doing?
2. What do you like to do the most?
3. What do you wish you were better at?
4. What talents do you have that you haven't developed?
5. Which of your skills are you most proud of? What do others most often say are your greatest strengths?
6. What have you gotten better at?
7. What can you just not get better at?
8. What do you most dislike doing?
9. Which skills do you need to develop to perform your job?
10. What sort of people do you work best/worst with?
11. What sort of organization brings out the best in you?
12. What were you doing when you were happiest in your work life?
13. What are your most cherished hopes for your future work life?

Source: Adapted from Hallowell, E. M. (2010, December). What brain science tells us about how to excel. *Harvard Business Review*, 126.

⊪ How Ambitious Are You?

1. I am able to put work out of my mind when off the job.

   True _____   False _____

2. I very much enjoy betting in football pools, lotteries, races, and so on.

   True _____   False _____

3. You only live once, so a happy life with many friends is more important than the hard work of attaining accomplishments.

   True _____   False _____

4. I very much dislike seeing things wasted (like food, fuel, paper, etc.).

   True _____   False _____

5. I make daily lists of things to do.

   True _____   False _____

Scoring: Give yourself 1 point for the following answers.

1. False
2. False
3. False
4. True
5. True

4–5 points: You are intensely ambitious.
2–3 points: You have an average level of ambition.
0–1 points: Your ambition level is low.

Source: Didato, S. V. (2003). *The big book of personality tests*. New York, NY: Black Dog and Leventhal, 102.

⊪ What's Your Pecuniary Profile?

Please answer the following questions:

1. To be rich means to be powerful.

   True _____   False _____

2. The bottom line is, money is the ultimate symbol of success.

   True _____   False _____

3. I like to buy top-of-the-line products.

   True _____   False _____

4. I often use money to persuade others to do what I want.

   True _____   False _____

5. When I discover that I earn more than someone I previously believed made more than I, I feel satisfied.

   True _____   False _____

Give yourself 1 point for each True response.

4–5 points: You believe money equals power and prestige.

2–3 points: You are average in your tendency to use money for power and prestige.

0–1 points: No matter how much money you have, you do not evaluate yourself or others based on their financial status.

Source: Didato, S. V. (2003). *The big book of personality tests*. New York, NY: Black Dog and Leventhal, 113.

Based on your responses, write a one-paragraph description of yourself as it relates to career.

⫶⫶⫶ Careers and the Emotional Intelligence Framework

Think about your mother and father. Have they ever discussed their careers, the career choices they made, and whether those choices worked out or made them happy? Do you think your parents have any career regrets?

Self-aware: Describe the best work experience you have ever had. What about it made it so? Can you relate this experience to career choices?

Self-management: Think about how you take feedback from your friends, family, coworkers, and employers. Is your attitude beneficial to you?

Social awareness: Who do you know that seems to be happiest in their job? Why is this?

Relationship management: If you have worked with or met a pharmacist who was cynical and burned out, how does this impact their interactions with other professionals and patients? Speculate as to why they are cynical or burned out.

⦙ Personal Learning Plan: Careers

These steps can be compiled on a single page containing the following:

> What prompted me to develop this plan?
>
> What is the general area for improvement?
>
> What is the specific issue for improvement?
>
> Why is this important to me?
>
> How do I generally act in these areas?
>
> What are my goals?
>
> What prompted this effort?
>
> What strategies are required?
>
> Who/what is necessary to meet my goals with this strategy?
>
> How will I measure the success/failure of this effort?
>
> How long will I focus on this effort?
>
> How will I reflect and capture a lesson from this effort that can be generalized to other circumstances?

⦙ WHAT'S IMPORTANT TO YOU IN THE CHAPTER?

With several of your classmates, discuss the idea/ideas that are most likely to effect change in your values, attitudes, or behaviors. Be succinct—no more than two sentences.

⦙ REFERENCES

Bushardt, S. C., Moore, R. N., & Debnath, S. C. (1982, Summer). Picking the right person for your mentor. *SAM Advanced Management Journal*, 46–51.

Didato, S. V. (2003). *The big book of personality tests*. New York, NY: Black Dog and Leventhal.

Hallowell, E. M. (2010, December). What brain science tells us about how to excel. *Harvard Business Review*, 123–129.

Kaplan, R. S. (2008, July–August). Reaching your potential. *Harvard Business Review*, 45–49.

Perez-Pena, R. (2012). Familiar faces offering advice, idealism and humor. *New York Times*. http://www.nytimes.com/2012/06/17us/graduation -speakers-offer-advice-idealism-and-humor.html?pagewanted=all.

⦚ SUGGESTED READINGS

Boyatzis, R., McKee, A., & Goleman, D. (2002, April). Reawakening your passion for work. *Harvard Business Review*, *80*(4), 87–94.

Donald, R. (2006). *Successful career management*. Bloomington, IN: Author House.

Groysberg, B., & Abrahams, R. (2010, January–February). Five ways to bungle a job change. *Harvard Business Review*, 137–140.

Ibarra, H. (2002, December). How to stay stuck in the wrong career. *Harvard Business Review*, 40–47.

Jackman, J. M., & Strober, M. H. (2003, April). Fear of feedback. *Harvard Business Review*, 101–107.

Janda, L. (1999). *Career tests*. Avon, MA: Adams Media.

Kocach, B. E. (2001). Successful derailment: What fast trackers can learn while they are off the track. *Organizational Dynamics*, *18*(2), 1833–47.

Kram, K. E. (1983). Phases of the mentor relationship. *Academy of Management Journal*, *26*(4), 608–625.

London, M. (1998). *Career barriers*. Mahwah, NJ: Lawrence Erlbaum Associates.

Miao, C. F., Lund, D. J., & Evans, K. R. (2009). Reexamining the influence of career stages on salesperson motivation; a cognitive and affective perspective. *Journal of Personal Selling and Sales Management*, *29*(3), 243–255.

Savage, L. M., Beall, J. W., & Woolley, T. W. (2009). Factors that influence the career goals of pharmacy students. *American Journal of Pharmacy Education*, *73*(2), 1–5.

Siracuse, M. V., Schondelmeyer, S. W., & Hadsall, R. S. (2004). Assessing career aspirations of pharmacy students. *American Journal of Pharmacy Education*, *68*(3), 1–12.

Stybel, L. J., & Peabody, M. (2001, July–August). The right way to be fired. *Harvard Business Review*, 87–95.

Super, D. E., & Hall, D. T. (1978). Career development: Exploration and planning. *Annual Review of Psychology*, *29*, 333–372.

CHAPTER 23

Difficult Conversations

Pre-Assessment: Difficult Conversations

Mind Mapping

Consider the terms arrayed on the page. For each term, without thinking or editing, write down the ideas, concepts, examples, contradictions, and theories that come to mind. Do not array them in any systematic or orderly manner. Scatter them about the page. Now, draw lines between your additions, indicating that there is a relationship between the terms. If something causes something else, indicate this with an arrow. Relationships may be reciprocal—both cause each other—requiring arrows at both ends. Indicate the strength of the relationship by darkening and thickening the lines; stronger relationships have darker and thicker lines. Most important: There is no right answer. Do not compare with your classmates. *What you have is a mind map, your mental representation of the topic. Review to determine if anything has changed following this section.*

Asking for a raise
Telling someone no
Confronting a coworker

⚜ DESIRED EDUCATIONAL OUTCOMES

- Discuss the structure of a difficult conversation.
- Demonstrate use of the scripting technique.

⚜ DESIRED PERSONAL OUTCOME

- Achieve greater facility in conducting a difficult conversation.

What Is the Underlying Structure of a Difficult Conversation?

ALMOST WITHOUT EXCEPTION, RESOLVING ANY problem at work comes down to having a conversation with someone. Often, such conversations can be unpleasant, difficult, and nonproductive. These conversations can be characterized as lobbing grenades. No matter how you coat it, or try to soften it, such conversations create noise and damage. Telling someone that their performance is not up to standard seldom happens without some collateral damage to individual relationships and attitudes towards the company. Although it is impossible to eliminate this aspect of a difficult conversation, it is possible to reduce the level of damage with practice and understanding.

All difficult conversations have an underlying structure consisting of three distinct aspects (adapted from Stone, Patton, & Heen, 1999):

- *The "What happened?" conversation:* Difficult conversations have an element of disagreement over what happened, didn't happen, or should have happened. It is the he said/she said aspect. Essentially, it is the attempt to determine who is right and who is to blame. The what happened conversation is grounded in three assumptions that cause problems: (1) I am right and you are wrong; (2) I assume I know your intentions; and (3) you are to blame.

- *The feelings conversation:* Typically, the feelings aspect of a difficult conversation is not revealed directly but through telltale remarks and asides. Comments such as, "This is the thanks I get?" signal hurt, whereas remarks about the amount of things that need to be done signal anxiety. The question is, what should we do with our feelings and emotions? Should we explicitly declare how we really feel?

Generally, most people opt for a "rational," businesslike approach in hopes of avoiding the messiness that feelings bring to the situation. However, difficult conversations don't just involve feelings; at their core they are about feelings. Not talking about feelings in these circumstances is like watching an opera without the score. You may get the plot, but will likely miss the point. The feelings part of a difficult conversation is clearly where the emotionally intelligent shine.

- *The identity conversation:* An aspect of a difficult conversation is the conversation we have with ourselves over what this situation means to us. It is an internal debate seeking to understand whether the claims against us are credible—whether we really are competent or to blame. Ultimately, the determination is whether we are loved or unloved. Even for the individual delivering unpleasant news in a difficult conversation, identity issues come into play: How is my self-esteem, my image of myself impacted by this conversation? I'm just asking for a raise, what does it mean about me if I don't get it? I always like to help people, what does it mean about me if I have to turn down a request for a raise from a competent employee due to budget constraints? The identity issue of a difficult conversation is the most subtle and may be the most challenging aspect of a difficult conversation.

What's the Secret to a Difficult Conversation?

THE RECOMMENDATIONS FOR HANDLING A difficult conversation follow from the problems related to each of the three aspects of difficult conversations. They are: let your assumptions go about intention and who is right or wrong; deal with feelings in an appropriate manner for the context; and consider the impact that such conversations have on your sense of who you are.

The Scripting Technique

A BENEFICIAL TECHNIQUE FOR DEALING WITH a difficult conversation is to script out the likely flow of the conversation; in other words, sit down and write out the possible courses that a difficult conversation could take (see Figure 23.1). Generally, such conversations move along three tracks. The first, and the one you hope for, is that when an individual is confronted with something he or she agrees with you and you mutually work out a resolution. The second is emotional—anger, resentment, hostility, and the like. The third is denial or resistance. Having considered the various responses prior to the meeting, it is less likely you will be caught unawares and that the conversation will not accomplish its intended objectives.

Some general rules for difficult conversations and scripting include:

- Take control of the situation by your choice of words and actions; set the tone for a professional discussion.

- Make a specific, direct request for what you want at some point in the conversation.

- Recognize that in most circumstances you have some power; let the other person know this without resorting to saying it. Never threaten.

- Never show your anger while deflecting and absorbing the other person's anger. Resorting to anger means you have lost; give the other person a chance to save face.

- Try to have the last word by expressing thanks, asking for reconsideration, or asking for another meeting.

Reducing Stress in a Difficult Conversation

A CONVERSATION IS NOT A VERBAL joust; it is not a contest to score points. It is about accomplishing an objective, conveying information, improving performance, clearing the air, and so on. Most people do not like participating in these conversations. The stress of such conversations can be reduced by first being clear in what you say. Euphemisms and talking in circles just confuse people and increase uncertainty. Being clear is not being brutal. Tone, facial expression, and body language determine how the content is perceived. The objective in this regard is neutrality. Think about how NASA communicates, no matter how dire the circumstances: "Houston, we have a problem." Finally, choose temperate phrasing and avoid inflammatory language, challenges, or lines in the sand. In such conversations, emotions are often close to the surface. Choosing inflammatory language may be the spark that ignites a fire.

Difficult Conversations at Work

THE FOLLOWING IS A SAMPLE scenario related to a difficult conversation involving RPG (recent pharmacy graduate):

> RPG didn't really like the intern, but she felt sorry for him. One night when it was slow the intern began to discuss his family situation. His brother had become addicted to drugs as an adolescent and had been in and out of treatment several times. His parents had exhausted all their resources providing rehabilitation, paying legal bills, and supporting the intern's brother. The intern revealed that his parents had just declared bankruptcy and that as they approached their retirement would not have any assets to support themselves. She also knew that the intern was financing his education without any help and that this job was important to him. The intern had an "edge"; he gave off an aura of repressed anger. Now, it was no longer repressed. When RPG came to work on Monday the time clock was off the wall and sitting on the floor. Apparently, the intern had gotten angry at closing time last Saturday and ripped the time clock off the wall.
>
> RPG knew she had to call the intern in to discuss the matter. She also knew that if he admitted the incident, she would have to fire him. She began to think about the conversation.

How would you recommend RPG handle the situation?

Assignment: What Do the Practitioners/ Others Say?

BE PREPARED TO DISCUSS DIFFICULT conversations based on any *one* of the following:

- A discussion with your colleagues on difficult conversations
- An article on difficult conversations, from either the research literature or any other source

- A movie/television program/YouTube video about difficult conversations
- A book on difficult conversations (literary, historical, psychological, or any other source)

EXERCISES

⍦ Responding to a Salary Offer

Figure 23.1 shows the various directions a conversation about salary can take. Refer to the scripted conversation as you work with several of your classmates on the scripts for the following scenarios:

Asking for a salary increase

Asking for a promotion

Ending a personal relationship

Asking your spouse to lose weight

Tactfully suggesting better hygiene to a subordinate

Confronting a backstabbing peer

Based on your responses, write a one-paragraph description of yourself as it relates to difficult conversations.

⍦ Difficult Conversations and the Emotional Intelligence Framework

As a professional, a clinician, and a supervisor, avoiding uncomfortable and difficult conversations will be impossible. Consider such conversations from an emotional intelligence framework.

Self-aware: List and describe your emotions when involved in a difficult conversation.

Self-management: How do you manage these circumstances? Do you avoid them? What do you tell yourself?

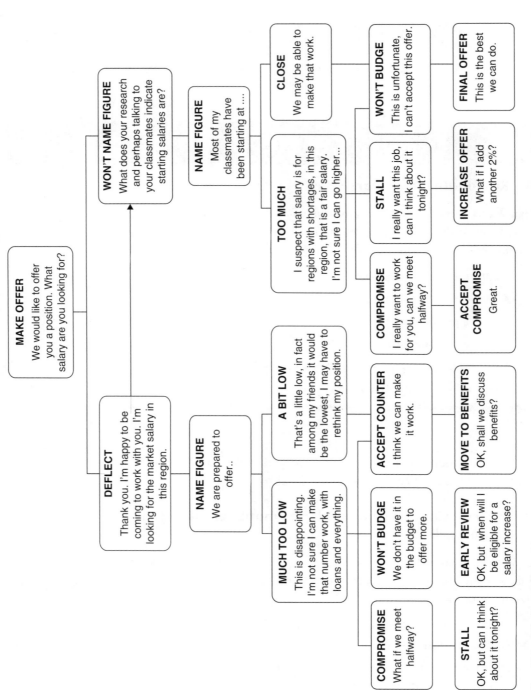

Figure 23.1   Difficult conversation script.

Social awareness: Do you know someone who is good at these types of conversations? If so, what do they do? If not, is there a character from television or the movies you can emulate in this regard?

Relationship management: What is the secret to having a difficult conversation and still maintaining or strengthening the relationship?

⫸ Personal Learning Plan: Difficult Conversations

These steps can be compiled on a single page containing the following:

What prompted me to develop this plan?

What is the general area for improvement?

What is the specific issue for improvement?

Why is this important to me?

How do I generally act in these areas?

What are my goals?

What prompted this effort?

What strategies are required?

Who/what is necessary to meet my goals with this strategy?

How will I measure the success/failure of this effort?

How long will I focus on this effort?

How will I reflect and capture a lesson from this effort that can be generalized to other circumstances?

⫸ WHAT'S IMPORTANT TO YOU IN THE CHAPTER?

With several of your classmates, discuss the idea/ideas that are most likely to effect change in your values, attitudes, or behaviors. Be succinct—no more than two sentences.

◆ SUGGESTED READINGS

Benjamin, S. F. (2008). *Perfect phrases for dealing with difficult people.* New York, NY: McGraw-Hill.

Lown, B. A. (2007). Difficult conversations: Anger in the clinician-patient/family relationship. *Southern Medical Journal, 100*(1), 34–39.

Pollan, S. M., & Levine, M. (1996). *Lifescripts.* Indianapolis, IN: Wiley.

Stone, D., Patton, B., & Heen, S. (1999). *Difficult conversations.* New York, NY: Penguin.

Weeks, H. (2001, July–August). Taking the stress out of stressful conversations. *Harvard Business Review*, 112–119.

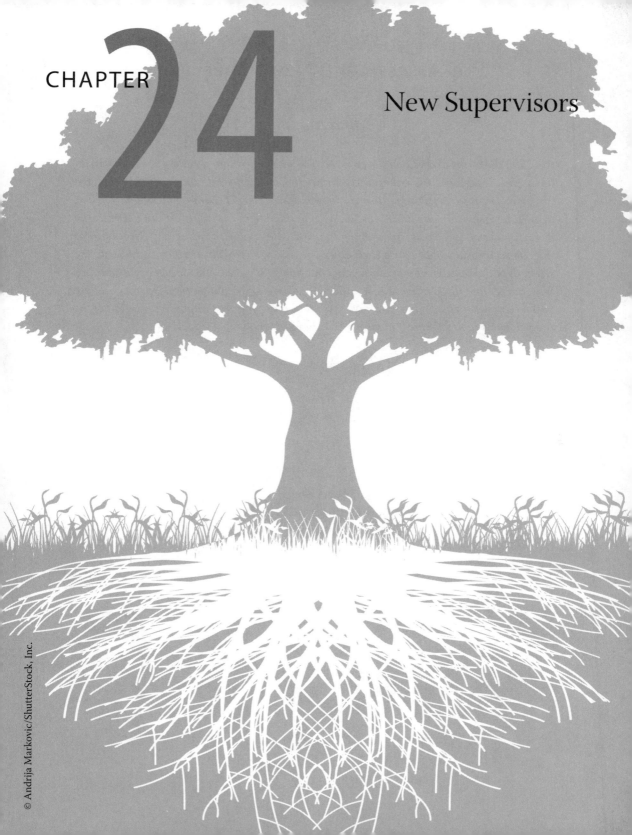

CHAPTER

24

New Supervisors

© Andrija Markovic/ShutterStock, Inc.

Pre-Assessment: New Supervisors

Mind Mapping

Consider the terms arrayed on the page. For each term, without thinking or editing, write down the ideas, concepts, examples, contradictions, and theories that come to mind. Do not array them in any systematic or orderly manner. Scatter them about the page. Now, draw lines between your additions, indicating that there is a relationship between the terms. If something causes something else, indicate this with an arrow. Relationships may be reciprocal—both cause each other—requiring arrows at both ends. Indicate the strength of the relationship by darkening and thickening the lines; stronger relationships have darker and thicker lines. Most important: There is no right answer. Do not compare with your classmates. *What you have is a mind map, your mental representation of the topic. Review to determine if anything has changed following this section.*

Supervisor
Supervisor tasks

⍾ **DESIRED EDUCATIONAL OUTCOMES**

- Describe what supervisors do.
- Describe mistakes supervisors tend to make.

⍾ **DESIRED PERSONAL OUTCOME**

- Succeed in your role as a supervisor.

Pharmacists as Supervisors

Not all pharmacists will be pharmacy managers. Not all pharmacists want or aspire to this role. However, all pharmacists, whether they want to or not, will act as supervisors. Let me repeat this statement for emphasis: all pharmacists will act as supervisors. Any time you as a pharmacist are working with technicians, or are tasked with making sure that specific activities occur, you are acting as a supervisor. There is no grace period for assuming this role following graduation. Supervision is part of the job. It is part of being a clinician. It is part of taking care of the patient.

What Do Supervisors Do?

Supervisors are front line managers, interacting directly and intimately with those doing the actual work. This is in contrast to middle managers and top management, who are relatively distant from the actual work of the department. As a front line supervisor you will still be expected to engage in the basic activities of the department—distribution, counseling, compounding, and so on; in other words, patient care. Coupled with these activities is the obligation to guide and direct the work of others. If the supervisory role is more formalized, then you will be concerned with staffing, budgeting, performance appraisal, hiring, firing, and the like. In this capacity, you will be acting as a manager. As already mentioned, the first day you are left alone following licensure, and you have technicians working with you, you are a supervisor.

A supervisor takes a group of people and attempts to direct, govern, control, and inspire them to accomplish the goals and objectives of the department. Why is this so hard? As the historian Barbara Tuchman (1981, p. 255) noted,

> The human being is unreliable as a scientific factor. In combination of personality, circumstance, and historical moment, each man is a package of variables impossible to duplicate. His birth, his parents, his siblings, his food, his home, his school, his economic and social status, his first job, his first girl, and the variables inherent in all of these, make up that mysterious compendium, personality—which then combines with another set of variables: country, climate, time, and historical circumstance. In short, people are unpredictable.

Supervision is not a science. Successful actions one day result in different and unwanted responses the next. Some aspects of supervision may result in relative standardization, but not absolute certainty. Sometimes supervision requires an "eye," a "feel," intuition, judgment, and attention to your gut. Sometimes you have to know when to break the rules, or establish new rules. It is this aspect of supervision that often troubles practitioners shaped by the rigor and relative certainty of science. The English writer G. K. Chesterton called life a "trap for logicians" because it is almost but not quite reasonable. "It just looks a little more mathematical and regular than it is. Its exactitude is obvious, but its inexactitude is hidden; its wildness lies in wait."

As a supervisor, in addition to responsibilities for clinical outcomes, you will be responsible for levels of customer service and operational efficiencies—waiting time, quality, units produced per unit of time, and so on. Each of these aspects impacts revenues, cash flows, margins, and profits. The difficulty is maintaining the appropriate balance among clinical outcomes, customer service, and efficiency metrics. It is the challenge of the position. Those above you may applaud your effort, but will only reward your performance. There is no *A* for effort.

Two Guidelines for Supervisors

AS YOUR CAREER PROGRESSES YOU will figure out, through experience, what works for you as a supervisor. Two ideas may be helpful initially as you develop your own methods.

- *Reciprocity drives human relationships.* It is unlikely that people will respond to you in a way that is different from the way that you treat them. This idea is linked to the concept of "you get what you expect." Treating people with courtesy, dignity, and respect will generally result in them treating you in the same way. This idea is particularly critical in a service business. If you want your employees to deliver superior service, you must give them superior service when they come to you with their problems. In general, an angry person won't continue to be angry in the face of your calm, reasonable response to them.

- *Do what works.* Despite what you read or believe constitutes good management or what good managers are supposed to do, the only effective guide is—do what works. If what you are doing is not working, get rid of it. The object is to win the game. Knowing and doing are not the same thing. Being able to analyze a case, identify a problem, or recite a correct answer is not the same as being able to effectively supervise.

What Mistakes Do New Supervisors Make?

ALMOST ALL NEW SUPERVISORS ARE prone to making two mistakes. The first tendency is for new supervisors to want the staff and employees to like them. Often, the staff and employees are contemporaries in age and experience. Often, they have shared the same work situations. In many cases they are your friends or drinking partners. Successful supervisors have to gain the respect and trust of the people they manage. The fact that you are a superior clinician with a great track record is not enough. Supervisors gain respect and trust by first demonstrating the content of their character. As a new supervisor, employees will read every gesture and comment to get a handle on who you are and how you will react in this role. Will you let the title go to your head? Will you consider your employees' feeling and concerns? Will it be about advancing their careers and aspirations, or yours? Will you ask them to do things that you wouldn't do yourself? On and on, like a farmer searches the sky for the nuances of the weather, employees search to get a handle on you, your style, and your patterns as a supervisor. Will the atmosphere at work be calm and professional or stormy, unpredictable, and chaotic?

The second tendency is the need to overcontrol. In the desire to perform, particularly in a pharmacy, new supervisors watch everything and want all decisions to come through them to make sure there are no mistakes. Very quickly it should become apparent that no one individual can watch and manage every detail and transaction. This is particularly true if the supervisory role is in addition to the responsibilities associated with distributive and clinical functions. New supervisors need to understand that their job is not to do the actual work but to build a team that will accomplish organizational objectives. Rather than building relations with individuals one at a time, the necessity is to forge a collective mentality and a sense of group that is focused on the task. Rather than watching every transaction, the successful supervisor is monitoring the group and assessing the overall performance.

Box 24.1   What Faulty Assumptions Do New Supervisors Hold?

Many of the problems that confront new supervisors are due to the faulty assumptions they hold, for example:

Myth: Now I will have the freedom to implement my ideas.

Reality: It's humbling that someone who works for me can get me fired.

Myth: I will finally be at the top of the ladder.

Reality: Everything but all the power, you have to earn their respect.

Myth: I must get compliance from my subordinates.

Reality: Compliance does not equal commitment.

Myth: My role is to build relationships with individual subordinates.

Reality: I need to create a culture that will allow the group to fulfill its potential.

Myth: My job is to make sure the operation runs smoothly.

Reality: I am responsible for initiating changes to enhance the group's performance.

Source: Adapted from Hill, L. A. (2007, January). Becoming the boss. *Harvard Business Review*, 51.

Supervision: The Primary Task

THE SUPERVISOR'S PRIMARY TASK IS to set the mood in the pharmacy. Think of how the atmosphere varies across the classes you have taken. In some classes time flies, whereas in others time is an eternity. Some classes are interesting, others sleep inducing. If you have worked in various pharmacies, or for different companies, think about how the mood varies in each one, whether it is fun to go to work, or a dread; whether time passes quickly, or drags. The variable that determines the mood in a classroom is the instructor; at work, it is the supervisor. Your task as a supervisor is to assess your own emotions and mood, make sure they are appropriate for the context of work, and then signal that mood to others. The ideal is a mood, or atmosphere, that makes work enjoyable while ensuring maximum productivity and clinical effectiveness.

Supervision at Work

THE FOLLOWING IS A SAMPLE scenario related to supervision involving RPG (recent pharmacy graduate):

RPG loved her new job. It was with a major health network hospital in a city she loved. Her colleagues were all first rate. As long as she stayed at the hospital she knew she would be on the cutting edge of practice. As a new hire, RPG was required to cover the night shift for a week once a month for the first year. At night she would be the only pharmacist in the 350-bed hospital. She also would have one technician to help her. Having just passed the board 6 months ago, RPG knew she was relatively inexperienced, but in general felt she was competent to handle any situation that would come her way. Most nights the workflow was steady and uneventful.

This evening was different. Everything seemed to be going wrong, and for some reason all the staff in the hospital seemed irritated. RPG turned to the technician and asked her to go to the floor and exchange an IV bag that the nurses had almost let run out. Time was running out to make the switch. When asked to go the floor, the technician looked RPG in the eye and declared, "You go get it, I'm going on break." RPG was flabbergasted. She knew she couldn't go, because other orders were coming into the pharmacy that required her attention. One of the nurses from the floor offered to come down and make the switch, so the immediate problem was solved. RPG still had to deal with the technician—once she got back from break.

How would you recommend RPG handle the situation?

Assignment: What Do the Practitioners/Others Say?

BE PREPARED TO DISCUSS NEW supervisors based on any *one* of the following:

- A discussion with your colleagues on their experiences as a new supervisor
- An article on new supervisors, from either the research literature or any other source
- A movie/television program/YouTube video about new supervisors
- A book on new supervisors (literary, historical, psychological, or any other source)

EXERCISES

⚜ **Would You Be an Understanding Boss?**

1. Men enjoy their jobs more than women do.

   True _____   False _____

2. If a worker is dissatisfied he or she will produce less.

   True _____   False _____

3. Job satisfaction tends to increase with age.

   True _____   False _____

4. Men tend to rely on their supervisors for job satisfaction more than women do.

   True _____   False _____

5. New employees tend to show high job satisfaction.

   True _____   False _____

6. Increasing workers' salaries improves their level of job contentment most of the time.

   True _____   False _____

7. Compared with high performers, low performers will do better if you provide them more chances to socialize on the job.

   True _____   False _____

8. The more intelligent a worker, the more satisfied he or she tends to be.

   True _____   False _____

9. Job dissatisfaction tends to increase with a worker's level of responsibility.

   True _____   False _____

10. Hours and work conditions are generally not important factors in job satisfaction.

   True _____   False _____

⑴⑾ Scoring

Give yourself 1 point for each response that matches yours.

1. False; 2. False; 3. False; 4. False; 5. False; 6. False; 7. True; 8. True; 9. False; 10. True

A score of 5 is average. A score above 5 indicates you have a better than average understanding of what makes workers happy.

Source: Didato, S. V. (2003). *The big book of personality tests*. New York, NY: Black Dog and Leventhal, 109.

Based on your responses, write a one-paragraph description of yourself as it relates to supervision.

⑴⑾ Supervision and the Emotional Intelligence Framework

Please read the following scenario and consider your response from an emotional intelligence perspective. (This scenario is based on an actual event.)

⊷ The Story

Sitting at the stoplight on the way to work, at the top of the hill, MKS looked down at Larrimer Pharmacy where she worked. She looked over the small town of Steelville, by the Allegheny River on the edge of Pittsburgh. It was a run-down, dilapidated former mill town. Row houses and bars fronted the main streets. The best house in the city could be bought for $40,000. It looked as though the sun never shone on Steelville. It seemed to MKS that it was always cloudy on the way to work, or raining. The only buildings that reflected continued care and prosperity were the Catholic church, the funeral homes, and Larrimer Pharmacy.

Larrimer Pharmacy was a surprisingly successful business. Entering the front of the pharmacy was like stepping into a 1950s pharmacy—not much had changed in 60 years.

Business was steady in the retail side of the pharmacy, but clearly not growing. In the back, in the closed pharmacy where MKS worked, business was booming. Larrimer had contracts with two large nursing homes and was negotiating with other smaller homes. MKS attributed the success of Larrimer Pharmacy to Jackie, the nonpharmacist, third-generation family member to own the business. Jackie was smart and tough—a real piece of work, and a story for a later day. MKS winced as she thought about the night she set off the security alarm and had to call and wake Jackie.

Walking into the pharmacy, MKS spotted Dave. Dave's job description was a combination technician/driver. He was an interesting young man, having gone to college to pursue an engineering degree. In his second year in school he switched to theater and graduated with his degree. He is extremely creative, funny, and talented. He has that kind of video game boy, slacker look—slightly disheveled, bearded, sloppy haircut, mix and match clothes, soft and fast-food pudgy. He could be thought of as an anti-corporate, anti-preppy, anti-Tommy Hilfiger, Nautica, Gap, Polo kind of guy. He has a wry, cynical take on the world, as if he has just discovered that the world is not as it seems. Dave's family is personal friends with Jackie.

Some days Dave is very helpful in the pharmacy. Others he is a nightmare. Today was one of the latter days. The pharmacy operation was designed to run with one pharmacist, two technicians, and Dave to fill in when needed. The day started badly for MKS, the pharmacist on duty. Jennifer, a board-certified technician, called just as the store opened and said she would not be coming to work. Her mother, a diagnosed schizo-phrenic who was constantly in and out of the hospital, had been hoarding her medications. Jennifer's mother had tried to commit suicide last night. Jennifer was an industrious, single mother with a small baby and a derelict boyfriend who was trying to put herself through school. MKS liked Jennifer and was worried about her.

Everything that came through the pharmacy that day was a problem. The orders were incorrect, doses wrong, doctors unavailable, nurses irri-table. It seemed for every new order, the pharmacy was out of the drug or the wholesaler had shorted the order. By 1 PM orders were about one hour delayed from what they would normally be. It looked like MKS would have to stay an extra hour to finish everything. This was not something MKS wanted to do because she was supposed to meet a new person for a drink, someone she liked and was hoping to develop into a relationship. Plus, MKS wanted to make it to the mall and have a few minutes to shop for her mother's Christmas present.

MKS asked Dave to pull the Zithromax from the shelf. For a few moments Dave broke into a splendid chorus of "It's a Small World" rendered in perfect tones and with theatrical flourish. A few pirouettes through the pharmacy, a bow, and a thank you completed the performance, quite good and entertaining. Dave started to pull the Zithromax from the shelf this way. He went to the "A" section of the shelves and started,

"A, it's not here."

"B, it's not here."

"C, it's not here."

Apparently, Dave planned to go through the alphabet. MKS had just drifted to the mean side of hungry. She thought, what is this about?

Self-aware: Describe the emotions that this circumstance arouses in you. Please list the actual emotions you think you would feel, not what you think you *should* feel.

Self-management: Describe how you would handle these emotions.

Social awareness: List one or two theories that might explain Dave's behavior.

Relationship management: How would you handle this situation?

◆ **Personal Learning Plan: Supervision**

These steps can be compiled on a single page containing the following:

> What prompted me to develop this plan?
>
> What is the general area for improvement?
>
> What is the specific issue for improvement?
>
> Why is this important to me?
>
> How do I generally act in these areas?
>
> What are my goals?
>
> What prompted this effort?
>
> What strategies are required?
>
> Who/what is necessary to meet my goals with this strategy?
>
> How will I measure the success/failure of this effort?
>
> How long will I focus on this effort?
>
> How will I reflect and capture a lesson from this effort that can be generalized to other circumstances?

◆ WHAT'S IMPORTANT TO YOU IN THE CHAPTER?

With several of your classmates. discuss the idea/ideas that are most likely to effect change in your values, attitudes, or behaviors. Be succinct—no more than two sentences.

◆ REFERENCES

Didato, S. V. (2003). *The big book of personality tests.* New York, NY: Black Dog and Leventhal.

Hill, L. A. (2007, January). Becoming the boss. *Harvard Business Review,* 49–56.

Tuchman, B. (1981). Is history a guide to the future? In *Practicing History: Selected Essays* (pp. 247–255). New York: Ballantine Books.

⫸ SUGGESTED READINGS

Goleman, D., Boyatzis, R., & McKee, A. (2001, December). Primal leadership: The hidden driver of performance. *Harvard Business Review*, 43–51.

Kramer, R. M. (2009, June). Rethinking trust. *Harvard Business Review*, 69–77.

McConnell, C. R. (2012). *The effective health care supervisor* (7th ed.). Burlington, MA: Jones and Bartlett.

Robbins, S. P., & DeCenzo, D. A. (2004). *Supervision today.* Upper Saddle River, NJ: Pearson Prentice Hall.

Stettner, M. (2000). *Skills for new managers.* New York, NY: McGraw-Hill.

Walker, C. A. (2002, April). Saving your rookie managers from themselves. *Harvard Business Review*, 3–7.

Politics

Pre-Assessment: Politics

Mind Mapping

Consider the terms arrayed on the page. For each term, without thinking or editing, write down the ideas, concepts, examples, contradictions, and theories that come to mind. Do not array them in any systematic or orderly manner. Scatter them about the page. Now, draw lines between your additions, indicating that there is a relationship between the terms. If something causes something else, indicate this with an arrow. Relationships may be reciprocal—both cause each other—requiring arrows at both ends. Indicate the strength of the relationship by darkening and thickening the lines; stronger relationships have darker and thicker lines. Most important: There is no right answer. Do not compare with your classmates. *What you have is a mind map, your mental representation of the topic. Review to determine if anything has changed following this section.*

Politics at work
Gossip at work
Ethics at work

⊯ DESIRED EDUCATIONAL OUTCOMES

- Consider the facts of organizational life.
- Discuss emotional intelligence and politics.
- Discuss gossip at work.
- Describe how to recognize a toxic work environment.

⊯ DESIRED PERSONAL OUTCOME

- Achieve greater skill at playing the political game at work.

You can wish all you want, but the facts in Box 25.1 are the rules by which the game of work is played. You can choose to compete to win this game, or operate as a martyr constantly sacrificing your interests, or remain clueless to the political impact of your behaviors, or operate as an amoral rogue player. The choice is yours.

Why Is There Politics at Work?

POLITICS IS NOT THE MARK of an aberrant organization. It is the mark of all organizations. In an ideal world politics at work wouldn't exist. Trust and harmony would abound. The focus would be on building a successful organization, maximizing health outcomes, and facilitating the personal growth and development of all concerned. Unfortunately, this

Box 25.1   What Are Some Facts of Organizational Life?

Organizations have their own rules. Here are some facts of organizational life:

- ❑ Organizations are not democracies.
- ❑ Some people have more power than others.
- ❑ All decisions are subjective.
- ❑ Your boss has significant power over your life.
- ❑ Fairness is not necessarily an organization goal.
- ❑ All organizations are somewhat dysfunctional, somewhat neurotic.

Source: Adapted from McIntyre, M. G. (2005). *Secrets to winning at office politics*. New York, NY: St. Martin's Griffin, 26.

is rarely the case when at work. Factions exist. There is competition for resources. Coalitions form to thwart other groups. Some people don't like one another. All people have relative levels of neurotic and dysfunctional behaviors that play out in the ongoing theater of work. Some will see your competence as an asset to the business, others as a threat to their position. At the extreme, politics at work can be debilitating. Generally, most organizations function reasonably well in spite of it. The point is that although you might lament the politics of work, if you want to be effective and survive and prosper at work, it is helpful to understand how to play the political game. Some examples of political tactics are (adapted from Zanzi & O'Neill, 2001):

- Exchanging favors
- Manipulating others
- Forming coalitions
- Persuasion
- Networking
- Ingratiation
- Providing resources

How Does Emotional Intelligence Help with Politics?

ALL ASPECTS OF EMOTIONAL INTELLIGENCE lend themselves to competing in the political game at work. Self-awareness lets you understand how you are perceived by others and who your natural allies, confidants, and mentors might be. Self-management lets you thrive under pressure without retaliating against those who might be out to sabotage your efforts. Social awareness lets you read the cues and understand what the hidden agenda might be regarding an issue. Relationship management lets you build social networks in order to be effective. It needs to be emphasized that most workplaces are relatively pleasant and appealing places to work. But it is the rare work environment that is not political.

What Is Prudent Paranoia?

IN TITLING THIS SECTION WE are not considering paranoia in the pathological clinical sense. Rather, the posture one should take is one of prudent suspicion. Acting from a perspective of prudent paranoia means one monitors the activities of associates, analyzes the subtext of meetings and conversations, checks for the rise and fall of one's status and reputation, and tries to understand who is in power, who is gaining power, and whose power is slipping away. In short, the prudently paranoid is a keen and penetrating observer of the social environment in which they work. The prudently paranoid person understands that something is always going on that may affect them. Think of an iceberg floating across the ocean. Only a small part is visible above the water line; the bulk of the iceberg is hidden, and it is that part that sunk the Titanic. The prudently paranoid trusts the dealer, but cuts the cards anyway (Kramer, 2002).

What Are the Unspoken Rules of Work?

ORGANIZATIONS HAVE FORMAL CHARTS INDICATING where power is located and the various reporting relationships. Implicit in these charts is the formula for how things should get done. In other words, for this problem I should check here; it will need to be reviewed by this committee, and ultimately win the approval of this individual. In addition to these formal charts, there is a shadow organizational framework for how things really get done. Even though the formal chart says to go here, the politically astute player understands how things really get decided. For example, you need to know that the executive assistant to the financial officer is the key to a decision because unless she is favorable to your point, she will bury your proposal. Or, if you really need a response from human resources the assistant director is the one to see, because the director is just marking time until retirement. Finally, the pharmacist in charge is the CEO's nephew and his job is secure no matter what his level of performance. In other words, you need to learn the unspoken and unwritten rules of the workplace.

What Is Power, and How Do I Use It?

Politics is ultimately about power and influence. Many people are ambivalent about the exercise of power. Without power nothing can be accomplished. The grand accomplishments of any organization are because one person, or several people, had the power to get things done. The appropriate exercise of power is a good and necessary thing. Our view of power is often shaded by our agreement with the ends for which it was used.

It is highly unlikely that a pharmacy student or a recent graduate will have much power. In this case, the task is to try to influence outcomes without having any authority. A range of tactics to influence others without formal authority include (adapted from Baldwin, Bommer, & Rubin, 2008):

- *Rational persuasion:* Using logical arguments and facts to persuade someone

- *Consultation:* Seeking someone's participation in developing something to win their support

- *Inspirational appeal:* Appealing to values, ideals, and aspirations to create enthusiasm

- *Ingratiation:* Getting someone in a good mood

- *Personal appeal:* Appealing to someone's loyalty or friendship

- *Exchange:* Offering to exchange favors

- *Coalition:* Seeking the help of other people, or using the support of other people to get someone to agree with you

- *Legitimizing:* Appealing to authority or pointing out consistency with existing norms or values

- *Pressure:* Using demands or threats

Of these nine choices, by far the most effective are an inspirational appeal, consultation, and a personal appeal; the least effective are legitimizing and pressure.

In playing the political game it is good not to discount the simple power of people liking you, for whatever reason—your personal attractiveness, your pleasant demeanor, your self-deprecating humor, or your resemblance to them. It is simply easier to get things from people if they are your friends. When you couple likeability with reciprocity (supporting others, being generous with time and expertise, doing the little things that need to be done) you have a powerful combination for organizational success.

Grapevines and Gossip

ALL WORKPLACES HAVE INFORMAL NETWORKS or "grapevines" that convey information, back stories, gossip, and rumors. Some of this information will be accurate; most will be fabricated or shaded for personal gain. It is important to make sure that you are hooked into this network. Typically, the grapevine is more interested in negative information about people and events. At work, one should assume there are no secrets. Anything you tell another person is not likely to be kept secret. Very few people are absolutely discreet about everything. Consequently, anything you say negative about a coworker is likely to make its way to them, often inaccurately conveyed. If you can't say something complimentary about a coworker, subordinate, or superior, the best advice is to say nothing at all. Gossip has the power to tarnish, or even ruin, people's careers. Information and innuendo spread by gossip is power. Rest assured that if a colleague is spreading gossip about someone else, they are also spreading gossip about you. Absorb all the information you can about the people and issues at work, but let it die with you.

Are There Ethics in Organizational Politics?

ORGANIZATIONS ARE ABOUT ACCOMPLISHING OBJECTIVES. Successful careers are about meeting personal objectives. However, that does not mean that any action can be justified as long as it furthers either organizational objectives or personal careers. There are acceptable rules to the political game. There are sanctioned and nonsanctioned activities. Examples of sanctioned political tactics include use of expertise, networking, coalition building, persuasion, image building, and superordinate goals (generating support by linking proposals to the greater good of the organization).

Examples of nonsanctioned political tactics include intimidation and innuendo, manipulation, control of information, blaming and attacking others, organizational placement (controlling promotion and assignment), co-optation (merging with another group or individual to silence them), and using surrogates (working through others). At the extreme, sabotage, mutinies, and duplicity are not acceptable. The political golden rule is this: "Never advance your own interests by harming the business or hurting other people" (McIntyre, 2005, p. 17).

How Do I Recognize a Toxic Political Environment?

SOME ORGANIZATIONS ARE CRIPPLED BY a malicious and toxic political landscape. Such places are to be avoided; if already there, then leaving is warranted. A toxic political environment is characterized by the following (adapted from MacIntyre, 2005, p. 103):

- Power plays and power struggles predominate.
- Management egos need to be stroked constantly.
- Management is only focused on taking care of themselves.
- Entire departments are at war with one another.
- Time is spent on covering yourself rather than organizational objectives.
- Gossip and backbiting predominate.
- Disagreements are personal.

Politics at Work

THE FOLLOWING IS A SAMPLE scenario related to politics involving RPG (recent pharmacy graduate):

Many of the senior staff were disillusioned with the current director of pharmacy. Over lunch, several senior pharmacists were advocating going over the director's head to the chief of operations for the hospital. RPG was aware that this was going on and recognized the potential career implications in handling this situation. RPG believed that although the current director was not the best he had ever worked with, RPG was not clear that going over the director's head was warranted. RPG considered how to "play" this situation. Not supporting the senior staff had implications, particularly if someone from this group were to be named the new director. Even if this didn't happen, RPG had to work with these people and recognized that their recommendations were considered when promotions were made. However, if RPG joined with this group in approaching senior hospital administration and there was a rebuff, RPG knew that the director would find out, with the attendant career implications. Issues like this were seldom secret. RPG personally liked everyone involved. Though risky, RPG was determined to stay neutral in this circumstance, neither endorsing nor siding with either side. The risk in this case was alienating both sides. As a relatively young practitioner, RPG decided to portray himself as not really having the expertise to judge the director's performance, and would let the formal administrative structure deal with this. To RPG this seemed the best choice.

How would you recommend RPG handle the situation?

Assignment: What Do the Practitioners/Others Say?

BE PREPARED TO DISCUSS POLITICS at work based on any *one* of the following:

- A discussion with your colleagues on politics at work

- An article on politics at work, from either the research literature or any other source

- A movie/television program/YouTube video about politics at work

- A book on politics at work (literary, historical, psychological, or any other source)

EXERCISES

⊪ Allies and Enemies

Take a moment to list your allies and enemies at work. List those people you consider to be allies, those who are neutral toward you, and those who are likely to be enemies. In thinking of your adversaries, further categorize them based on this scheme:

Focused adversaries: Others who want to get their way, and see you as an impediment.

Emotional adversaries: Others who are out of control due to their emotional needs; their behaviors are often dysfunctional and rooted in anger and anxiety.

Vengeful adversaries: Others who are out to get you, either overtly or quietly. These people are vicious.

Source: Adapted from McIntyre, M. G. (2005). *Secrets to winning at office politics.* New York, NY: St. Martin's Griffin, 63–66.

⊪ Coalitions

Consider people at work as members of coalitions, groups of people who have the same interests and tend to act in concert. What is the basis of their mutual interest? For example, older male pharmacists close to retirement who do not have a Doctor of Pharmacy degree are a likely coalition.

Coalition One:_____

Basis for Coalition: _____

Coalition Two: _____

Basis for Coalition: _____

Coalition Three: _____

Basis for Coalition: _____

⫶⊪ Networks

Begin with a copy of the formal organization chart where you work. Construct an advice network by determining who specific people would go to for advice. For example, who does the associate director go to for advice? The point is, not who they are supposed to go to for advice, but who do they actually go to? Similarly, construct a trust network. For example, who does the associate director trust with work-related concerns?

Source: Krackhardt, D., & Hanson, J. R. (1993, July–August). Informal networks: The company. *Harvard Business Review*, 107.

⫶⊪ Political Skills Inventory

Take a few moments to reflect on how much you agree with these comments.

- I spend a lot of time and effort at work networking with others.
- At work, I know a lot of important people and I am well connected.
- It is important that people believe I am sincere in what I say and do.
- When communicating with others, I try to be genuine in what I say and do.
- I always seem to instinctively know the right thing to say or do to influence others.
- I have good intuition or savvy about how to present myself to others.
- It is easy for me to develop good rapport with most people.
- I am able to make most people feel comfortable and at ease around me.

Source: Vigoda-Gadot, E., & Meisier, G. (2010, January/February). Emotions in management and the management of emotions: The impact of emotional intelligence and organizational politics on public sector employees. *Public Administration Review*, 84.

⫶⊪ What Does This Mean?

Former President Lyndon Johnson said the following about FBI Director J. Edgar Hoover: "It's probably better to have him inside the tent pissing out, than outside the tent pissing in."

What does this mean regarding enemies and politics at work?

Based on your responses, write a one-paragraph description of yourself as it relates to politics.

⫸ Politics and the Emotional Intelligence Framework

If you want to be successful at work, understanding the political game is a must. Take a few moments to consider the following:

Self-aware: Do you relish the "messiness" of organizational politics, or do you find it draining and a waste of time?

Self-management: Can you keep a secret at work?

Social awareness: Who is your biggest enemy at work? Why is this so?

Relationship management: Is there any way to convert your biggest enemy at work into an ally?

⫸ Personal Learning Plan: Politics

These steps can be compiled on a single page containing the following:

What prompted me to develop this plan?

What is the general area for improvement?

What is the specific issue for improvement?

Why is this important to me?

How do I generally act in these areas?

What are my goals?

What prompted this effort?

What strategies are required?

Who/what is necessary to meet my goals with this strategy?

How will I measure the success/failure of this effort?

How long will I focus on this effort?

How will I reflect and capture a lesson from this effort that can be generalized to other circumstances?

⚜ WHAT'S IMPORTANT TO YOU IN THE CHAPTER?

With several of your classmates, discuss the idea/ideas that are most likely to effect change in your values, attitudes, or behaviors. Be succinct—no more than two sentences.

⚜ REFERENCES

Baldwin, T. T., Bommer, W. H., & Rubin, R. S. (2008). *Developing management skills*. New York, NY: McGraw-Hill Irwin.

Krackhardt, D., & Hanson, J. R. (1993, July–August). Informal networks: The company. *Harvard Business Review*, 104–111.

Kramer, R. M. (2002, July). When paranoia makes sense. *Harvard Business Review*, 62–69.

McIntyre, M. G. (2005). *Secrets to winning at office politics*. New York, NY: St. Martin's Griffin.

Vigoda-Gadot, E., & Meisier, G. (2010, January/February). Emotions in management and the management of emotions: The impact of emotional intelligence and organizational politics on public sector employees. *Public Administration Review*, 72–86.

Zanzi, A., & O'Neill, R. M. (2001). Sanctioned versus non-sanctioned political tactics. *Journal of Management Issues, 13*(2), 245–262.

⚜ SUGGESTED READINGS

Buchanan, D. A. (2008). You stab my back, I'll stab yours: Management experience and perceptions of organization political behavior. *British Journal of Management, 19*, 49–64.

Farrell, D., & Petersen, J. C. (1982). Patterns of political behavior in organizations. *Academy of Management Review, 7*(3), 403–412.

Kurland, N. B., & Pelled, L. H. (2000). Passing the word: Toward a model of gossip and power in the workplace. *Academy of Management Review, 25*(2), 428–438.

Zaleznik, A. (1997, November–December). Real work. *Harvard Business Review*, 53–62.

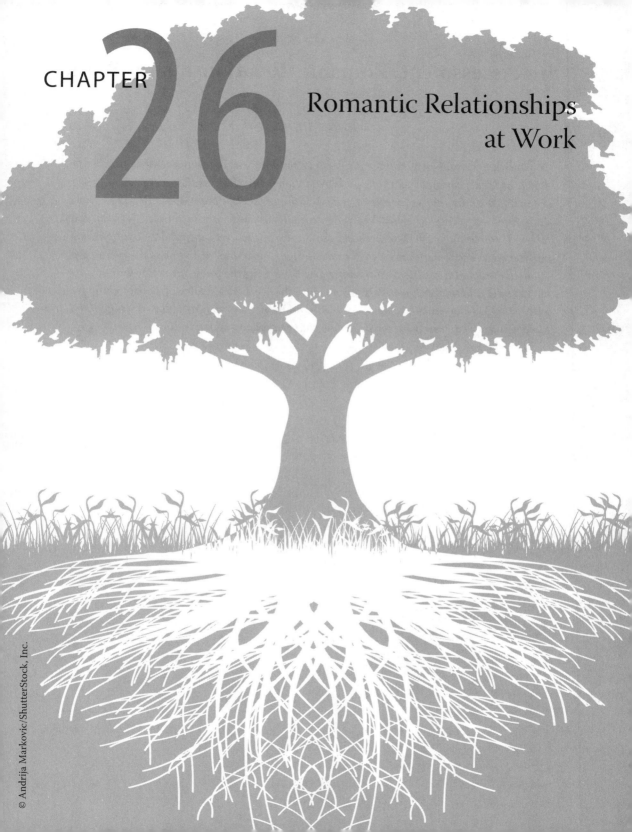

CHAPTER

26

Romantic Relationships
at Work

Pre-Assessment: Romantic Relationships at Work

Mind Mapping

Consider the terms arrayed on the page. For each term, without thinking or editing, write down the ideas, concepts, examples, contradictions, and theories that come to mind. Do not array them in any systematic or orderly manner. Scatter them about the page. Now, draw lines between your additions, indicating that there is a relationship between the terms. If something causes something else, indicate this with an arrow. Relationships may be reciprocal—both cause each other—requiring arrows at both ends. Indicate the strength of the relationship by darkening and thickening the lines; stronger relationships have darker and thicker lines. Most important: There is no right answer. Do not compare with your classmates. *What you have is a mind map, your mental representation of the topic. Review to determine if anything has changed following this section.*

Dating at work
Flirting at work
Sexuality at work

〰 DESIRED EDUCATIONAL OUTCOME

- Discuss the issues related to romantic relationships at work.

〰 DESIRED PERSONAL OUTCOME

- Understand appropriate, professional, and ethical behavior in this aspect of work.

Are Romantic Relationships Inevitable?

TODAY, MOST PHARMACISTS WORK IN larger practice settings than before. This is in contrast to a generation ago, where much of practice was in smaller organizations, typically with only two or three other people. For new practitioners in their twenties it is hardly surprising that issues related to finding and establishing personal relationships occupy much of their energy. This discussion recognizes that you simply cannot control human behavior and the human heart.

Our focus is on romantic relationships that are voluntary on the part of both people and have no societal or ethical sanctions or impediments attached; that is, both people are single and available with no coercion or significant power differences. In other words, there is no hint of sexual harassment or quid pro quo—they are consensual relationships. Our interest is in romantic relationships that do not violate a specific corporate policy.

Is This a Legal Issue?

IN GENERAL, COMPANIES HAVE A right to promulgate rules and regulations regarding dating at work. However, this right has to be balanced with the employee's right to privacy. Some companies adopt strict prohibitions against romantic involvement at work. Others adopt a policy that actively discourages these relationships, but nevertheless permits romantic involvements. Some organizations insist that those involved in romantic relationships inform their superiors. This option is problematic if the romantic relationship is same sex. Some companies have the parties to a romantic relationship sign a "love contract," essentially a document that eliminates the employer's liability. Finally, some companies avoid adopting any formal policy and rely on unwritten rules and cultural norms to handle each situation, generally forms of quiet persuasion. The key is to understand what the rules of the game are and act accordingly.

Failed romantic relationships create potential workplace issues with legal implications. If one party following the termination of a failed romantic relationship acts in a manner that is unacceptable, such acts may be construed as creating gender-based harassment rather than personal enmity. Supervisors should be cognizant of such situations and should ensure that remedial action is taken. Although one may feel angry or betrayed following a failed romantic relationship at work, it is not acceptable to act unprofessionally, or worse, outrageously.

As an employee, one should not assume that emails and Internet usage on company systems are private. Someone from the company may be reading your emails. In doing so, if they discover a romantic involvement in violation of company policy, or emails that are inappropriate in content or that contain derogatory comments regarding others at work, then action by the company may be forthcoming. Remember, don't put something in an email that you don't want others to read.

Are Romantic Relationships at Work Secret?

THE ANSWER TO THIS QUESTION is relatively simple and straightforward. No matter how discreet you believe you are, such relationships are seldom secret for very long. People will notice, with some being supportive and others jealous and condemning. People will look for issues of favoritism. People will look to see if the quantity and quality of work are impacted. People will want to know if their desires in the organization are being responded to equitably, or whether they are somehow compromised by this new relationship. It is difficult to maintain a professional relationship with someone you are romantically linked to. It is equally difficult to keep it secret.

What Happens When Romantic Relationships End?

THE ENDING OF A ROMANTIC relationship is fraught with peril. Suddenness and the desire of one person to end the relationship can result in a messy and prolonged separation stage. Just as it is difficult to maintain a professional relationship with someone you are enamored of, it might be more difficult to maintain a professional relationship with someone who has broken your heart. Consider 12-hour days next to a colleague pharmacist with whom you have just broken up. To say the least, it will be awkward. At the extreme, one partner's desire to maintain the relationship may become obsessive and disruptive.

The Illusion of a Romantic Relationship

THE ILLUSION OF A ROMANTIC relationship is an issue. Frequent or exclusive lunches together fuel the rumor mill and beget gossip. Such gossip, even if unfounded, may impact your reputation based on the supposition that many people believe where there is smoke there is fire. If there are issues with your performance, people may see this imagined relationship as contributory. There are no secrets at work. No matter how clandestine you believe you are, someone will pick up on the subtle cues. Be aware of this, and conduct yourself in a manner that does not compromise your professional reputation, your credibility, and more importantly your performance. There is very little you can do to silence the rumor mill other than to be conscious of how your behavior is perceived.

General Guidelines for Romantic Relationships at Work

THE FOLLOWING ARE SOME GUIDELINES on how to handle a romantic relationship at work professionally (adapted from Schaefer & Tudor, 2001):

- Conduct yourself as a professional. Be discrete and avoid public displays of affection.
- Do not take long lunches or breaks together. Avoid returning with a disheveled appearance.

- Love may be blind, your colleagues are not.
- Romantic relationships with clients, suppliers, and vendors create potential conflicts of interest.
- Asking someone for a date, if company policy allows, is acceptable. Overly aggressive persistence may constitute harassment.
- Do not call in sick on the same day.
- If working in an environment with international colleagues, recognize that different cultural norms may apply.

Sexuality and Sexual Humor at Work

SEXUAL BANTERING AND FLIRTING ARE commonplace at work, as is sexual humor. The issue is the distinction between these activities taking place with consensual agreements between willing parties and sexual harassment. Sexual harassment is against the law. Sexual bantering, flirting, and sexual humor may be illegal if they create an intimidating, hostile, or offensive environment. Comments acceptable to one person may be offensive to another. Comments at a certain time may be appropriate, whereas the same comments in a different context may be unacceptable. If you are the object of unwarranted attention or humor, the first recourse is to confront the individual directly and convey your objections. If this does not work, then going to a supervisor is appropriate. In health care, sexual bantering, flirting, and sexual humor may be used to reduce stress. Again, this may be appropriate or not, depending on the individuals and circumstances. It is important to remember the following: be aware of the norms of the workplace, evaluate the potential risk to your career, and be sensitive to the reactions of people when engaged in these behaviors.

Romantic Relationships at Work

THE FOLLOWING IS A SAMPLE scenario related to romantic relationships involving RPG (recent pharmacy graduate):

RPG is 26 years old and graduated from pharmacy school 2 years ago. He is single and unattached. Currently he is working at a major medical center in an urban area. His responsibilities are divided between the customary dispensing roles and clinical involvement on the floor, though his clinical involvement is gradually increasing due to his clearly recognized gift for this activity. Every 5 weeks, seven new sixth-year pharmacy students are assigned to the hospital for their clinical rotations. Approximately half of RPG's time is spent on the floor with several of the students. This cohort contains five women and two men. RPG is clearly attracted to one of the female students, and in their initial encounters it seems that she is attracted to him. RPG has noticed that in clinical meetings the female student makes it a point to sit by him and seems particularly eager to consult with him regarding patients on the floor and her projects. RPG will be involved in assigning grades for these students. At lunch last week the female student made it known that she had just broken up with her fiancé. RPG took this as an opening to ask her out. RPG desperately wanted to invite her to join a group of practitioners that would often go to happy hour on Friday night. RPG was finding it hard to be impartial in his assessment of her performance and was somewhat reluctant to critique her performance. RPG began to recognize that these feelings and attitudes toward the student were unfair and on the verge of becoming unprofessional.

How would you recommend RPG handle the situation?

Assignment: What Do the Practitioners/Others Say?

B E PREPARED TO DISCUSS ROMANTIC relationships at work based on any *one* of the following:

- A discussion with your colleagues on romantic relationships at work
- An article on romantic relationships at work, from either the research literature or any other source
- A movie/television program/YouTube video about romantic relationships at work
- A book on romantic relationships at work (literary, historical, psychological, or any other source)

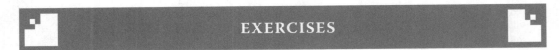

EXERCISES

Discuss with your classmates:

- What is appropriate flirtation at work, if any?

- What is appropriate in asking someone to go out? How persistent should you be?

- Does overt sexuality have a place at work? Have you seen colleagues at work use their sexuality to their advantage?

- Do people perceive these relationships differently if they believe it is the beginning of an enduring relationship, or just a fling?

- Have you observed any workplace romances? How did the people involved handle it? Were they appropriate? What were the consequences of their relationship?

- Have you observed any nontraditional romantic relationships at work? How did the people involved handle it? Were they appropriate? What were the consequences of their relationship?

Based on your responses, write a one-paragraph description of yourself as it relates to romantic relationships at work.

⚬ Romantic Relationships at Work and the Emotional Intelligence Framework

Attraction and romantic relationships are inevitable at work. Understanding how to deal with these circumstances is important to a career and to acting as a professional. At the extreme, they may compromise patient care if those involved are inordinately focused on one another at the expense of the patient.

Self-aware: Have you ever been physically attracted to someone at work? Describe the feelings.

Self-management: What tactics did you use to manage these feelings? If you have not had this experience, what would you recommend as the appropriate way to manage these feelings?

Social awareness: How can you tell if someone is romantically interested in another person?

Relationship management: If you have been attracted to someone at work, how did you handle the relationship? How have you seen others at work handle these situations?

Personal Learning Plan: Romantic Relationships at Work

These steps can be compiled on a single page containing the following:

What prompted me to develop this plan?

What is the general area for improvement?

What is the specific issue for improvement?

Why is this important to me?

How do I generally act in these areas?

What are my goals?

What prompted this effort?

What strategies are required?

Who/what is necessary to meet my goals with this strategy?

How will I measure the success/failure of this effort?

How long will I focus on this effort?

How will I reflect and capture a lesson from this effort that can be generalized to other circumstances?

WHAT'S IMPORTANT TO YOU IN THE CHAPTER?

With several of your classmates, discuss the idea/ideas that are most likely to effect change in your values, attitudes, or behaviors. Be succinct—no more than two sentences.

⬩ REFERENCE

Schaefer, C. M., & Tudor, T. R. (2001). Managing workplace romances. *Advanced Management Journal*, 66(3), 4–10.

⬩ SUGGESTED READINGS

Arnesen, D. W., & Weis, S. L. (2007). Developing an effective company policy for employee Internet and email use. *Journal of Organizational Culture, Communication, and Conflict*, 11(2), 53–65.

Dowd, S., & Davidhizar, R. (2003). Sexuality, sexual harassment, and sexual humor. *Health Care Manager*, 22(2), 144–151.

Hovick, S. R. A., Meyers, R. A., & Timmerman, C. E. (2003). E-mail communications in workplace romantic relationships. *Communication Studies*, 54(4), 468–482.

Powell, G. N., & Foley, S. (1998). Something to talk about: Romantic relationships in organizational settings. *Journal of Management*, 24(3), 421–448.

Schultz, V. (2003). The sanitized workplace. *Yale Law Journal*, 112, 2061–2191.

Williams, C. L., Giuffre, P. A., & Dellinger, K. (1999). Sexuality in the workplace: Organizational control, sexual harassment, and the pursuit of pleasure. *Annual Review of Sociology*, 25, 73–93.

Wilson, R. J., Filosa, C., & Fennel A. (2003). Romantic relationships at work: Does privacy trump the dating police? *Defense Counsel Journal*, 70(1), 78–88.

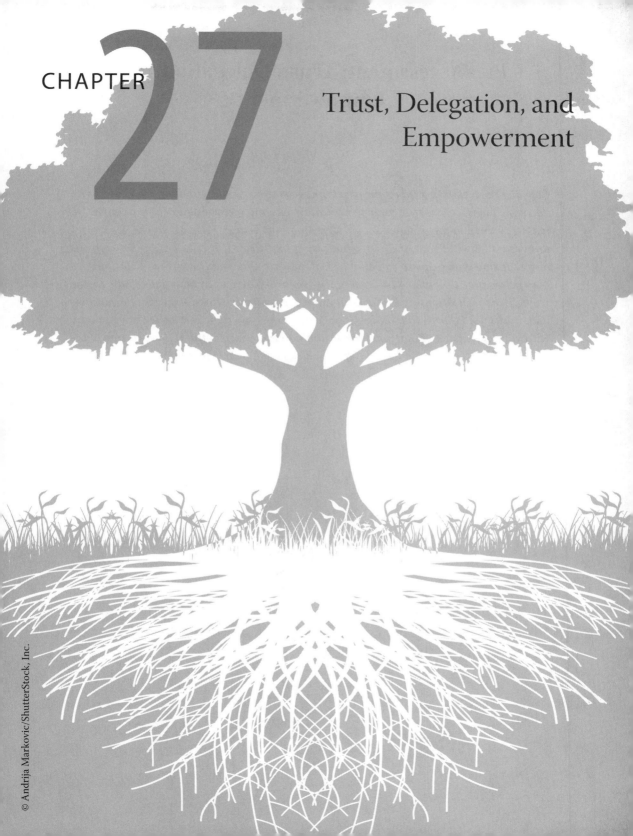

CHAPTER

27

Trust, Delegation, and Empowerment

Pre-Assessment: Trust, Delegation, and Empowerment

Mind Mapping

Consider the terms arrayed on the page. For each term, without thinking or editing, write down the ideas, concepts, examples, contradictions, and theories that come to mind. Do not array them in any systematic or orderly manner. Scatter them about the page. Now, draw lines between your additions, indicating that there is a relationship between the terms. If something causes something else, indicate this with an arrow. Relationships may be reciprocal—both cause each other—requiring arrows at both ends. Indicate the strength of the relationship by darkening and thickening the lines; stronger relationships have darker and thicker lines. Most important: There is no right answer. Do not compare with your classmates. *What you have is a mind map, your mental representation of the topic. Review to determine if anything has changed following this section.*

Trust
Delegation
Empowerment

◀ DESIRED EDUCATIONAL OUTCOMES

- Describe the mindsets related to trust.
- Discuss effective delegation.
- Discuss the benefits of delegation.

◀ DESIRED PERSONAL OUTCOME

- Use trust and delegation more effectively at work.

Trust

TRUST IS THE EXPECTANCY THAT an individual will keep their word or promise, that they can be relied on; it is a belief that someone else will protect your interests. Trust is fragile—years in the building, it can be expended with one act. Trust is a gamble. We decide to trust in the belief that the benefits of trusting outweigh the risks. Trust involves both emotions and cognitions. I have a good feeling about trusting you, or I believe you can be trusted.

To be human is to trust. Trust has value from an evolutionary perspective. For the most part, we conduct ourselves with a presumption of trust triggered by such simple things as a person who resembles us, a member of our group, or a simple touch on the shoulder. Although we may have a presumptive tendency to trust, often based on superficial cues, we can never completely assess another's motives or trustworthiness. In order to learn to trust, one needs to adjust their mindset and develop certain behavioral habits, including the following (Kramer, 2009):

- *Know yourself:* If you tend to trust the wrong people, work on reading the social cues people send regarding this matter. If you are good at reading people but find it difficult to forge relationships built on trust, then work on expanding your trust-building behaviors.

- *Start small:* Trust begins with small acts that are reciprocated.

- *Understand when not to trust:* Set the boundaries that will limit the extension of trust.

- *Send strong signals:* Signal that you are willing to trust and that you will retaliate if trust is abused.

- *Recognize the other person's dilemma:* Other people have the same fears about trusting us; understand and allay their fears.
- *Remain vigilant:* Due diligence in extending trust is required. Periodic checks to see if trust is still warranted are advised.

As a supervisor, trust is eroded by inconsistent messages, inconsistent standards, misplaced benevolence, false feedback, a failure to trust others, rumors, and a reluctance to confront painful and politically charged situations.

Trust is the matrix on which the effective operation of organizations and the healthcare system is arrayed. Without trust, effective delegation is impossible. The decision to trust at the individual, team, and organizational level is based on the following 10 elements (adapted from Hurley, 2012). Three of these elements relate to the trustor, and seven to the situation.

Trustor

- *Risk tolerance:* Faith that things will work out versus the need for assurance that they will.
- *Psychological adjustment:* How comfortable are you with yourself and the world?
- *Relative power:* Those high in power tend to trust more because they can punish transgressions, whereas those low in power do not trust as much because they have little recourse.

Situation

- *Security:* The higher the stakes, the less likely people will trust.
- *Similarities:* How much are people like you?
- *Alignment of interests:* To what degree are our objectives and interests aligned?
- *Benevolent concern:* Do we believe others will put our interests above theirs, or are they self-centered?
- *Capability:* Is the one we are trusting capable of fulfilling their promise?
- *Predictability and integrity:* How certain are we that they will carry out their promise? Do they overpromise and underdeliver?
- *Communication:* Is the communication open, honest, and frequent?

What Are the Characteristics of Effective Delegation?

DELEGATION HAS SEVERAL ASPECTS TO it. First, an allocation of specific duties and the assignment of responsibility for the task. Those delegated with a task must be given commensurate authority to accomplish the objective. Second, they must be held accountable for the objective. To whom should you delegate responsibility? Clearly, the answer is to those individuals who are capable of accomplishing the task, or those individuals who have the potential to grow into the role through experience or coaching.

Why Do I Need to Delegate?

THE ADVANTAGES OF DELEGATION FOR the pharmacist are that it frees up time, enhances relationships, improves decisions, and develops subordinates. There are disadvantages to delegation in that it is slower and that there are likely to be mistakes. At the managerial level for pharmacists, it is impossible to administer and run any pharmacy without help via delegated responsibility. Consider the various tasks related to the management of a pharmacy: distribution, clinical responsibility and coordination, staffing, purchasing, billing, payments, and so on. No single individual can oversee all these tasks simultaneously, nor is any single individual likely to be the most proficient at all these functions. Delegation is a must.

Further, the issue of delegation is critical to the practitioner. Specifically, what aspects of practice will you delegate to technicians, interns, and clerks? In a busy pharmacy, no pharmacist in charge can oversee and intervene in all interactions with patients, other healthcare practitioners, family members, providers, and payors. Within the limits of the law, all practitioners have to work out their policy towards delegating the various aspects of practice. Without effective delegation the system would simply grind to a halt, and practitioners would quickly burn out.

Empowerment

A S A RESULT OF THIS delegation, it is hoped that an empowered employee emerges. Our definition of an empowered employee is one who treats the organization as if he or she were one of the owners. Acting as if they were an owner, an empowered employee is motivated to protect the long-term interests of the organization and is committed to its betterment and survival.

The ideas of trust, delegation, and empowerment at work are grounded in two basic recognitions. One is easy to understand—no single individual can do all the work themselves. The second may require alterations in attitude and may not be quite as obvious as the first, but it is no less true—you are not the smartest person in the room.

Trust, Delegation, and Empowerment at Work

T HE FOLLOWING ARE SAMPLE SCENARIOS related to trust, delegation, and empowerment involving RPG (recent pharmacy graduate):

> RPG recognized that work flow in the pharmacy would be improved if he could delegate more of the routine tasks to a recently hired technician. This technician had been hired by the director of pharmacy as an attempt to elevate the level of customer service. In the past, RPG had delegated such tasks to technicians that he trusted. There was something about this technician that set off some ill-defined and hard to verbalize alarms for RPG. To RPG it seemed as if this technician had a hard time following through and was somewhat unfocused. One night RPG met one of his former classmates and began discussing work and this situation. It turns out that his former classmate and this technician were neighbors in the same condominium development. His classmate knew her to be a good neighbor and levelheaded, though he just heard that her twin sister was diagnosed with a terminal disease. RPG now had a confirmation for the feelings he was picking up about the technician, a confirmation for the validity of his intuition, and a confirmation of the value in paying attention to the behaviors and patterns of the people he worked with.

How would you recommend RPG handle the situation?

RPG found herself working in a high-volume chain pharmacy, usually about 700–800 prescriptions per day. As with all such operations, work was divided and orders moved through in an assembly line fashion. RPG began to consider the implications of her inputting orders with her name on them, but the orders then being filled and checked by others. In the event of a mistake, she would be the only one documented on the order.

How would you recommend RPG handle the situation?

Assignment: What Do the Practitioners/ Others Say?

BE PREPARED TO DISCUSS TRUST, delegation, and empowerment based on any *one* of the following:

- A discussion with your colleagues at work on trust, delegation, and empowerment

- An article on trust, or delegation, or empowerment from either the research literature or any other source

- A movie/television program/YouTube video about trust, or delegation, or empowerment

- A book on trust, or delegation, or empowerment (literary, historical, psychological, or any other source)

EXERCISES

Have you ever been betrayed in the past by a colleague, friend, or significant other? What did it feel like? What was the root cause of this betrayal? What did you miss in assessing this situation?

Beliefs About Human Nature

With your classmates, discuss whether you believe people are basically honest. Are there circumstances in which a basically decent person will lie, cheat, or steal?

⦚⦚ What Would You Delegate?

With your classmates, discuss the activities you would delegate to a person listed in the table. Do your choices vary from your classmates'? Are there circumstances in which you would allow someone to exceed their customary allowances? Would, for example, all technicians be allowed to do the same things, or would it vary by individual? How would you handle each category if they exceeded their level of autonomy?

Duties	Graduate Interns	Interns	Licensed Technicians	Technicians	Clerks

Based on your responses, write a one-paragraph description of yourself as it relates to trust, delegation, and empowerment.

⦚⦚ Trust and the Emotional Intelligence Framework

Have you ever been betrayed by a significant other, coworker, or fellow student? Recall the event and how it felt.

Self-aware: Determine if you trust too easily or don't trust at all. What are the potential implications of your approach to trust?

Self-management: How do you conduct yourself if you don't believe you can trust someone? Would you give someone a second chance if they betrayed you?

Social awareness: What markers indicate someone is an individual you can trust?

Relationship management: What is the appropriate level of trust in a personal relationship? A professional relationship?

⊪ Personal Learning Plan: Trust

These steps can be compiled on a single page containing the following:

What prompted me to develop this plan?

What is the general area for improvement?

What is the specific issue for improvement?

Why is this important to me?

How do I generally act in these areas?

What are my goals?

What prompted this effort?

What strategies are required?

Who/what is necessary to meet my goals with this strategy?

How will I measure the success/failure of this effort?

How long will I focus on this effort?

How will I reflect and capture a lesson from this effort that can be generalized to other circumstances?

⊪ WHAT'S IMPORTANT TO YOU IN THE CHAPTER?

With several of your classmates, discuss the idea/ideas that are most likely to effect change in your values, attitudes, or behaviors. Be succinct—no more than two sentences.

⊪ REFERENCES

Hurley, R. F. (2012). *The decision to trust.* San Francisco, CA: Jossey-Bass.
Kramer, R. M. (2009, June). Rethinking trust. *Harvard Business Review,* 69–77.

❖ SUGGESTED READINGS

Berg, J., Dickhaut, J., & McCabe, K. (1995). Trust, reciprocity, and social history. *Games and Economic Behavior, 10*(1), 122–142.

Covey, S. M. R., & Merrill, R. R. (2006). *The speed of trust.* New York, NY: Free Press.

Galford, R., & Drapeau, A. S. (2003, February). The enemies of trust. *Harvard Business Review,* 1–7.

Gilson, L. (2006). Trust in health care: Theoretical perspectives and research needs. *Journal of Health Organization and Management, 20*(5), 359–375.

Hurley, R. F. (2006, September). The decision to trust. *Harvard Business Review,* 55–62.

Kelly, P., & Marthaler, M. T. (2011). *Nursing delegation, setting priorities, and making patient care assignments.* Clifton Park, NY: Delmar Cengage Learning.

Wrightsman, L. S. (1964). Measurement of philosophies of human nature. *Psychological Reports, 14,* 743–751.

CHAPTER 28

Practical Advice

MOST LIKELY, YOU WILL SPEND a third of the rest of your life at work. Although it may not seem so now, work that is productive and fulfilling, with a group of people you like and admire, in an organization tasked with improving the lives of others is critical to a happy life. This is not to say that work won't have its frustrations and disappointments—it will. Your experience at work is, for the most part, a function of your behavior. What follows are some practical suggestions for improving that experience. These rules for work apply across all circumstances.

Personal responsibility: You are in charge; no one else makes you feel or do anything. Excuses are just that—an excuse for not doing something. Although many people will applaud your effort, in general, they will only reward your performance. As one writer suggests, "Your success is your own damn fault." Although you must take credit for your setbacks, you can also take credit for your successes.

Luck: Poker players say that over the short run luck may prevail, but over time skill guarantees winning. Every once in a while in life you may be able to skate by, but over time, preparation, work, and dedication are the only things that ensure success. It has been suggested that luck is the "residue of design."

Don't confuse simple with easy: Many things in life are easy to understand, but hard to do. Just because something sounds simple doesn't mean you can do it. Crafting a vision, creating a positive culture at work, motivating a tech, and using good clinical judgment are all tasks that can be understood easily; doing them well and consistently is another thing.

Never go over someone's head: Think about it—how would you like someone challenging your authority by going to your boss. Organizations establish reporting relationships for a reason, so honor them. Only two circumstances warrant violating this caution: if your superior is doing something that is either illegal or grossly unethical.

Stop whining: No one wants to hear it. If you need to, do it with your nonprofessional friends, after hours. Better yet, tell the dog. Everyone has their own problems. Energy spent whining can be better spent just fixing the problem.

Everyone is neurotic, including you: It is easy to see it in other people— their little eccentricities of attitude and behavior, their slightly skewed take on life, work, and relationships. The Chinese say that it is impossible to see your own eyelash, meaning it's difficult to see your own peculiarities; they are too close. You are neurotic like everyone else; you are just used to your own quirks.

Take the high road: If you don't know how to handle a situation, the fallback advice is to always take the high road. The fact that someone else is immature or petty does not require you to stoop to that level. Taking the high road is often the difficult choice. You might even come off looking second best by doing so, for now. The long-term benefit for this choice may not be apparent, but it is there nevertheless; you just can't see it slightly over the horizon.

Put things into perspective: Most problems at work and in life are relatively minor, sometimes even trivial. The basketball coach Al McGuire said you only needed to win two things, war and surgery. Confronted with a work situation, ask yourself, "Is anyone going to die?" If not, don't get too worried. If you don't believe this is true, think about this: how important today is the test that you got an 88 on rather than the expected 96, or the date who stood you up sophomore year in high school? In short, no matter what happens, the world will continue to spin.

People are not out to get you . . . they are, however, looking out for themselves: It is helpful not to see people at work as enemies. They are rivals, and like you they are seeking advancement, awards, and recognition. Impute as high a motive to your coworkers' behaviors as you do for your own.

If it doesn't work, try something else: A lot of situations at work don't have easy or right answers. If the approach you are now using isn't working, discard it. There are no points for style or method, only results. There are very few absolute commandments at work.

Look for the simplest solutions: If someone has trouble getting to work on time, ask him or her why before you develop an elaborate tracking system.

Keep things private as long as you can: Almost without exception, the way to handle any situation at work, at least initially, is privately and outside the formal mechanisms. Once memos and emails get sent, the organization has to initiate its often heavy-handed response. Very few problems require a zero tolerance attitude. Situations handled in private allow people the wiggle room often required to save face.

Organizations are not rational places: Organizations are made up of people. Neither people nor organizations are rational. People and organizations do stupid things; both engage in self-handicapping behaviors and both get in the way of themselves. All organizations have their inexplicable Catch-22 that doesn't make sense. You just have to accept this fact.

Friends at work: People at work are not your friends. They are your professional colleagues. There is a difference. An appropriate amount of distance and circumspection in dealing with people at work is warranted.

Finally, at the end of your life, the only things you will get to keep will be the things you have given away, in other words, the good you have done. This is the measure of a true professional.

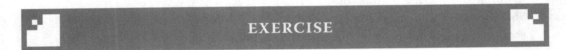

EXERCISE

Discuss with your classmates and colleagues at work whether they can add to this list of practical advice.

IV

Commandments at Work

At the end of each chapter you were asked to list what was important to you in that chapter. Collect the statements for each chapter and review. Can any statements be combined, eliminated, or synthesized into simpler and more personally useful statements? The task is to arrive at the fewest statements that capture the essence of what is important and memorable. In other words, what are you likely to remember in 6 months or a year? Consult with your classmates on this exercise.

◆ WHAT'S IMPORTANT TO YOU IN THE CHAPTER?

The Boss:

Careers:

Difficult Conversations:

New Supervisors:

Politics:

Romantic Relationships at Work:

Trust, Delegation, and Empowerment:

Glossary

Abuse of power: Using power for reasons other than the betterment of the patient and society, typically for personal gain

Accountability: The obligation of one party to be held responsible for its actions by another interested party

Achievement motivation: The personal striving of individuals to attain goals

Altruism: Seeking to increase the welfare of another person rather than yourself

Andragogy: The art and science of helping adults learn

Arrogance: An offensive display of superiority and self-importance resulting in haughtiness, vanity, insolence, and disdain

Attribution theory: How people justify their performance decisions; how people explain their behavior

Autonomy: The ability to make one's own decisions

Beneficence: Doing good

Bullying: A form of aggression; a repeated, unwelcomed negative act or acts (physical, verbal, or psychological intimidation) that can involve criticism and humiliation intended to cause fear, distress, or harm

Burnout: The loss of idealism, energy, and purpose in which mental and physical resources are gradually depleted

Career barrier: The brick walls that get in the way of fulfilling your career aspirations

Character: The foundation of conduct; an expression of the values and sensibilities of an individual

Cognitive reappraisal: Changing how you think about something

Compassion: The ability to notice the suffering of another

Compassion fatigue: The emotional, physical, social, and spiritual exhaustion that overtakes a person and causes a pervasive decline in his or her desire, ability, and energy to feel and care for others

Complex emotions: Emotions with multiple layers and sources

Conflict of interest: When the interest of the professional is placed above the interest of the patient

Conscientiousness: A global personality measure; fulfilling responsibilities

Consummate professional: Someone who conducts him- or herself professionally in all circumstances

Cultural intelligence: The ability to accommodate variation in people and circumstances arising from cultural differences

Dark side: Nonprofessional behaviors and traits

Delegation: Allocation of specific duties and the assignment of responsibility for a task along with commensurate authority

Difficult conversation: A conversation that can be unpleasant, difficult, and nonproductive

Duty: The free acceptance of a commitment to service

Emotion: A feeling and its cognitive, physiological, and behavioral components

Emotional addiction: Familiar emotional reactions and patterns we can't control

Emotional blinders: Excessive emotions that cloud our judgment, blinding us to social cues in the environment

Emotional hijackings: Circumstances, people, or objects that provoke uncontrolled emotional reactions

Emotional intelligence: The ability to understand your emotions, as well as others' emotions, and to craft a functional behavior suitable to the context

Emotional labor: A requirement that the practitioner display and regulate his or her emotions to fit the circumstances

Emotional regulation: The process and strategies by which individuals modulate their emotions

Empathy: The ability to understand and appreciate how another person feels

Empowerment: Feelings by an employee focused on protecting the long-term interests of the organization and its betterment

Entitlement: An expectation of success without a personal responsibility for achieving that success

Excellence: A conscientious effort to exceed ordinary expectations

Expertise: High levels of skills, knowledge, or abilities

Fear and anxiety: Normal reactions to potentially threatening events, either real or imagined

Fidelity: Faithfulness to duty or obligation

Flow: The sensation that people feel when they act with total involvement; when time seems to fly; being motivated by the task itself

Greed: When money becomes the driving force; an inordinate pursuit of power, fame, and money

Guilt: Feelings arising from violating a standard including remorse, anxiety, and regret at having done something to hurt someone else; focuses on the act

Honor and integrity: The consistent regard for the highest standards of behavior and the refusal to violate one's personal and professional codes

Impairment: Diminished capacity as a result of alcohol, drugs, or mental state

Incivility: Behaviors that are rude and discourteous

Intuition: Occurs outside of conscious thought; a holistic and integrating associative process; the subconscious application of previous learning to a current situation; automated expertise

Judgment: The ability to infer, estimate, and predict the character of unknown events

Justice: Fair and equal treatment

Machiavellianism: Manipulation for personal gain; elevating expediency over principle

Mentor: Someone you learn from at work and who helps advance your career

Misrepresentation: Lying and fraud; lying is consciously failing to tell the truth; fraud is a conscious misrepresentation of fact intended to mislead

Moods: Emotions that are muted but persist for an extended period (a day or two)

Moral intelligence: Using emotions to make ethical decisions and act on them

Moral reasoning: The ability to filter values, attitudes, emotions, and behaviors into good and evil

Narcissism: An inflated view of the self and fantasies of control, admiration, and success

Nonmaleficence: Doing no harm

Pedagogy: The art and science of teaching children

Personal learning plan: Formal statement of a self-directed exercise in learning

Person-centeredness: A view that values people as individuals

Politics: The human side of getting things done at work

Power: The ability to influence someone to do something

Practical intelligence: The pragmatic know-how to get things done

Primary emotions: Emotions that are hard-wired into the human central nervous system

Profession: An occupation characterized by mastery of a body of knowledge, high levels of autonomy, a code of behavior, and a social contract to do good for the individual and society

Professional: Anyone who adheres to the standards of a profession and practices within that profession

Professionalism: A complex pattern of values, attitudes, and behaviors reflecting the standards of the profession

Prudent paranoia: Wary suspicion of what is going on at work and how it might affect you

Psychopathy: A lack of concern for others and the rules of society; a lack of guilt; a clinical disorder rather than a personality trait

Reciprocity: The idea that other people react to you based on how you treat them

Relationship management: The delicate balance between doing things to preserve the relationship and doing things to preserve personal integrity

Respect for others: Humanism; understanding that a person, no matter his or her status, conditions, or accomplishments, is entitled to a standard of treatment

Rudeness: To disregard another; to diminish and demean; to invalidate the worth of another

Schema: How a person thinks about the world and him- or herself; a theory of how people and the world work

Self-awareness: The ability to understand who you are; an accurate picture of one's self and an understanding of how one behaves

Self-concept: The picture of ourselves based on the internalized set of perceptions we have made regarding ourselves

Self-control: Altering behaviors to conform to a standard

Self-directed learning: Learning devised and conducted by an individual

Self-efficacy: The belief that one can cope with adversity and accomplish difficult or novel tasks; the belief that you can do the job

Self-forgiveness: Acting benevolently toward oneself rather than punishing; eliminating feelings of self-hatred and self-contempt

Self-management: What you do, or do not do, that is appropriate to the context

Self-observation: The act of paying attention to ourselves dispassionately, without criticism or evaluation

Self-talk: The inner monologue or dialogue that goes on in our brain

Sensitive line: The point where information about ourselves is painful; the point we defend psychologically

Shame: Feelings of inadequacy, self-contempt, embarrassment, self-exposure, and indignity; shame focuses on the self

Simple emotions: Emotions with a single source, unfettered by other circumstances

Social awareness: Paying attention to the people and the world around you; seeing people as they are, not as you would like them to be

Stress: The body's reaction to any demand

Stupidity: The learned corruption of learning; the unquestioning acceptance of any one set of constraints or axioms; not thinking

Successful relationship: People resonate with one another and both are willing to do the work to sustain the relationship

Supervision: Directing and guiding the work of others while still functioning as a clinician

Temperament: The tendency towards a specific mood over a very long time

Toxic political environment: Time is spent on winning the game of work rather than on accomplishing objectives

Toxic relationship: When you are asked to sacrifice all of your needs for the enrichment of the other person

Transference: The understanding that no relationship is new; all current relationships are colored by previous relationships

Trust: The expectancy that an individual will keep their word or promise

Values: Enduring beliefs of what is good or desirable

Veracity: Truthfulness

Virtue: Conforming to standards, rules, doctrines, and lessons that delineate right and wrong behavior

Willpower: Resisting temptation; controlling our moods, emotions, thoughts, and behavior in pursuit of performance

Wisdom: Tacit knowledge as mediated by values toward the goal of achieving a common good; understanding the essence of the human condition and the conduct of a good life; knowing what is important

Worry: The cognitive component of anxiety; the anxious apprehension of events

Index